Management of
Erectile Dysfunction
in Clinical Practice

Culley C. Carson
University of North Carolina, Chapel Hill, USA

John D. Dean
The Prostate Centre, London, UK

Management of Erectile Dysfunction in Clinical Practice

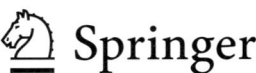 Springer

Culley C Carson, MD
Rhodes Distinguished Professor
Chief of Urology
Division of Urologic Surgery
University of North Carolina at Chapel Hill
Chapel Hill, NC, USA

Dr John D Dean, MBBS, FRCGP
Sexual Physician
The Prostate Centre
London, UK

British Library Cataloguing in Publication Data

A catalogue record for this book is available from the British Library

Library of Congress Control Number: 2006923492

ISBN-10: 1-84628-398-1   e-ISBN 1-84628-399-X   Printed on acid-free paper

ISBN-13: 978-1-84628-398-7

Springer Science+Business Media, LLC

springer.com

CONTENTS

AUTHOR BIOGRAPHIES

Professor Culley C Carson III, MD, is the Rhodes Distinguished Professor of Urology and Chief of Urology at the University of North Carolina Hospital, Chapel Hill, as well as Associate Chairman of the Department of Surgery at North Carolina School of Medicine, Chapel Hill. Previously, he served as a Director of the Duke Male Sexual Dysfunction Clinic, and is Consulting Urologist at several North Carolina hospitals. Professor Carson is currently the Editor-in-Chief of *Contemporary Urology* where he was awarded the 2001 Jesse H Neal Award for editorial writing, the Editor of *Mediguide to Urology*, Associate Editor of *Techniques in Urology*. He has published more than 200 peer review articles and eight textbooks. He is author of *Textbook of Erectile Dysfunction*, which was awarded the 2000 Book Prize by the Royal College of Medicine. Professor Carson is an active member of the American Association of Clinical Urologists, International Society for Impotence Research, American Association of Genitourinary Surgeons, American Surgical Association. Dr Carson serves as past president of the Sexual Medicine Society and president of the Southeast Section of the American Urologic Association. Professor Carson received his M.D. from the George Washington University School of Medicine in Washington, DC. He did his Surgical Residency at the Dartmouth-Hitchcock Medical Center and was a Urology Resident and Fellow at the Mayo Clinic in Rochester, Minnesota.

Dr John D Dean, MBBS, FRCGP, is a Sexual Physician, working in London and Devon, UK. Having originally trained as a Family Physician, he has provided care for men and women affected by sexual problems since 1985. He is interested in all aspects of both men's and women's sexuality, sexual endocrinology, gender identity disorders, and the ethics of sexual medicine. He has authored or co-authored over 60 publications, including books for health professionals on the management of erectile dysfunction in primary care, on sexual problems in general, on dyslipidemia and on medical education. He is Secretary-General of the European Society for Sexual Medicine, and a member of the European Association of Urology and of the International Society for the Study of Women's Sexual Health. He is also Chairman of the Ethics Committees of the *Journal of Sexual Medicine* and the International Society for the Study of Women's Sexual Health.

INTRODUCTION

Our understanding of, and attitude toward, male sexual health, and in particular, erectile function and dysfunction, is dynamic and has been continuously evolving. As recently as 25 years ago, this field was considered to be the exclusive domain of psychologists and/or endocrinologists. The advent of penile prosthesis insertion in 1973 and other, non-surgical, therapies such as vacuum constriction devices and local self-injection of agents in the 1980s brought the urologist to the forefront of clinical practice. This speciality has contributed greatly to current understanding of the physiology of the erectile process, the pathophysiology of erectile dysfunction (ED) and diagnostic and therapeutic options in patient management. Not surprisingly, from the therapeutic perspective alone, there has been, and continues to be, considerable improvement in the availability of user-friendly, reliable, and dependable interventions in the area of male sexual health.

Despite the prevalence of ED, up to the late 1990s fewer than one in ten men sought treatment for this disorder, and even within this subpopulation, a high treatment dropout rate was routinely observed [1]. Reasons advanced include the fact that treatment has been relatively invasive/intrusive in nature or artificial, has associated risks, may be irreversible, and is expensive. On this basis, it was anticipated that the general availability of the first effective oral agents, sildenafil, tadalafil and vardenafil, for the management of ED would have a considerable and far-reaching impact on the management of male sexual health issues. Certainly, there has been a major change in medical focus; primary care physicians have increasingly become the 'front line' in the management of patients complaining of sexual disorders. It is pertinent to note, however, that even with the arrival of the highly effective phosphodiesterase inhibitors the majority of men suffering from ED still do not present to discuss the condition with their physician [1].

With the advent of effective oral agents, the primary care physician has become the front line for ED management

Treatment
algorithms are
useful in facilitating
dialogue

The advent of more widespread awareness that ED is an important health problem, and the availability of orally active agents, have resulted in the requirement for accepted treatment algorithms to be used specifically as the potential basis for patient management in the community setting. The objective is to facilitate dialogue between physicians, patients and, increasingly, the initial healthcare provider in issues relating to male sexual health. One example, based on that developed by the *2nd International Consultation on Sexual Dysfunctions* [2], is shown in Figure 1.

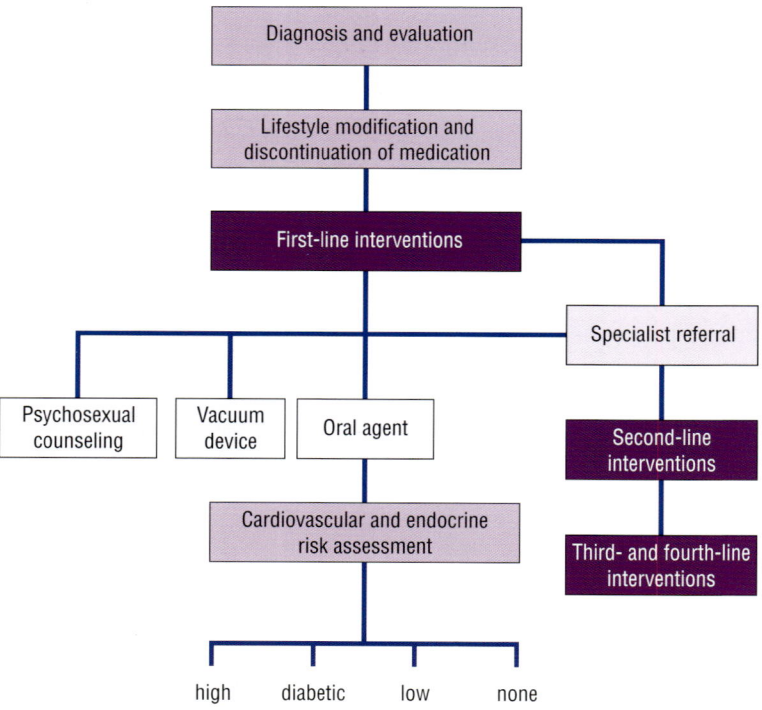

Figure 1. Treatment algorithm for management of ED patients

Why identifying and treating ED is an important primary care issue

Primary care is the ideal situation for health screening and promotion, as well as for the treatment of most chronic health problems. Family physicians will usually have detailed knowledge of the physical and psychological health of the individual, his partner and their family, and of their social context. This is often unavailable to the secondary care physician. As all of these factors have a particular bearing on sexual health, the family physician is ideally placed to assess and manage the majority of men with ED.

As well as the benefits to sufferers of being able to receive care from a trusted medical adviser, the physician may also benefit. Aside from the professional satisfaction derived from successfully managing a distressing condition and detecting a previously hidden health problem, there are benefits for the doctor–patient relationship. Because of the almost immediate benefits of modern ED therapies, the positive feedback from individuals and couples is most gratifying. Treating a man's hypertension for 10 years may prevent him from having a stroke, but he will not necessarily notice or acknowledge this. Enabling him to enjoy sexual intimacy again is quite a different matter.

Healthcare providers, economic planners and the public are concerned about the economic impact of the development of safe, effective and, therefore, widely used therapies for ED. In this context there are four major influences: *ED is highly prevalent, its incidence is age-related, it is a progressive condition, and it is currently significantly under-treated.*

The economic impact of a disease or medical condition is not limited to the cost of diagnosis and treatment. Various models are being used to determine the overall socio-economic cost of ED. *This includes lost time at work, decreased productivity, and effects on partner, family and co-workers.* Although

Unlike the secondary care physician, the family physician will usually have good knowledge of the health of the patient, his partner and their social context

The economics of ED extend beyond the cost of diagnosis and treatment

3

data gathering is incomplete, it is obvious that ED results in considerable indirect costs to society.

However, before it will be possible to predict the precise economic cost of ED, several key questions will have to be answered. These include:

- We know the cost of existing therapies, but how much will the rate of ED prescription increase with the introduction of new therapies in the future?
- What will be the average treatment duration?
- How many patients will progress from medical management to more invasive or expensive forms of intervention?
- What is the negative impact of the co-morbidities associated with ED (e.g. depression and decreased quality of life [QoL])?
- What is the positive impact of effectively managing co-morbidities identified in the ED assessment process?
- What is the positive impact of improving QoL?

Although it is only an estimate, prescription audits have shown that direct drug costs are already in excess of US$3 billion per annum. It is not unreasonable to assume that the indirect costs will be at least two to three times this figure, probably without even factoring in the additional cost to the primary care physician.

Direct costs of ED are already in excess of US$3 billion per annum and the indirect costs may be 2–3 times more

It is obvious that the economic impact of ED has increased significantly, since the introduction of sildenafil in the late 1990s, and will continue to grow at a substantial rate. The reasons for this increase are:

- Emerging patient population for this previously under-treated condition
- Introduction of phosphodiesterase type-5 (PDE5) inhibitors and other new therapies
- Increased ED awareness and education, secondary to direct consumer campaigns from the pharmaceutical industry

- The increasing prevalence of ED risk factors, such as diabetes and cardiovascular disease, in men in the developed world

Intimacy, sexuality, and ED as health issues

Intimate relationships are central to the human experience. We are, by nature, social creatures and, aside from a small minority of ascetics and hermits, we need each other's company. Without the ability to share intimate relationships, most of us will become isolated, lonely, anxious, and depressed.

Most people would not consider their life complete without sharing intimate relationships. Sexuality and sexual behavior are very important within the vast majority of those relationships.

The frequency of sexual feelings and behavior usually varies during the course of a relationship. Early on in a relationship, sex is relatively frequent, irrespective of whether the partners are young or old. This is may be a major concern for older men, in their 60s and 70s, when they begin a new relationship.

Physical intimacy plays an important part in developing the emotional intimacy that will later help the relationship endure over time. Throughout the course of the relationship, which may be 60 or more years, sex will become more or less important, and more or less frequent, at different times. It is, however, just as important to older couples as to younger couples, as one way of sharing the intimacy and closeness that will maintain their relationship.

Health is, according to the World Health Organization, a state of complete physical, psychological, and social well-being [2]. Without the ability to express ourselves through sexuality, and to form and maintain intimate relationships, we cannot achieve 'health'. As ED frequently interferes with that ability to form intimate relationships, as well as being a marker for major health problems, it clearly is a health issue.

ED frequently interferes with the ability to form and sustain intimate relationships

5

ED and sexual dysfunction as markers for other major health problems

Improving 'Men's Health' should be a major concern for all physicians. On average, a man's life expectancy is 7 years less than that of a woman [3]. They will often prematurely die, or become disabled by preventable diseases. This difference has traditionally been attributed to some unchangeable genetic susceptibility. However, the gap is slowly narrowing and the validity of this assumption is now highly questionable.

In the developed world, women have frequent contact with healthcare services throughout their lives, from the cradle to the grave. 'Women's Health' is perceived as a priority and access to it is considered an inviolable right for all women. After completing childhood health surveillance procedures, they will see a family physician regularly to obtain contraception, for ante-, peri- and post-natal care, for cervical cytology screening, for advice about the menopause and hormone replacement therapy, and for mammographic screening. They will also bring along their children and grandchildren for advice, providing further opportunities for health screening and advice.

Some men will not see a doctor from the time of their last childhood health surveillance consultation until they have their first heart attack, or worse. They often consider themselves 'immortal' and unable to spare the time for health maintenance. Any opportunity to encourage men to participate in health screening and maintenance activities should be enthusiastically developed by primary care teams.

Men *are* concerned about their sexual health and function. A minority of men with sexual problems (30–50%) seek professional advice [4]. Reasons for this include embarrassment, belief that ED is temporary or not important, and concern that the physician will not be interested [5]. The increased public awareness and acceptance of sexual problems that followed the development of oral therapies for ED is improving this situation

Some men will not see their doctor until their first coronary

Increased public awareness of sexual dysfunction has increased the likelihood of men to seek help

6

and, in the future, men are increasingly likely to ask their family physician for help.

ED is a symptom, not a disease. There are always underlying causes and it is clearly in the patient's best interest to seek them out. ED is strongly associated with a range of important, potentially life-shortening disorders, and may be the first presenting symptom of those disorders.

The association of ED with other disorders
It occurs in up to:

- 20% of men with untreated hypertension
- 45% of men with coronary artery disease
- 60% of men with diabetes
- 40% of men with chronic renal impairment
- 50% of men with chronic arthritis
- 63% of men with chronic alcoholism
- 80% of men with multiple sclerosis
- 70% of men with lower urinary tract symptoms (LUTS)
- 60% of men following treatment for prostate cancer

ED shares many of the same risk factors as coronary heart disease, including dyslipidemia, smoking, hypertension, diabetes, and sedentary lifestyle [1,6]. All men who complain of ED should be offered a thorough cardiovascular risk assessment, including screening for dyslipidemia, diabetes and hypertension.

ED should be considered a symptom, not a disease

Cardiovascular risk assessment should be considered for ED patients

Prevalence and incidence of ED

Although ED is considered to be a benign disorder it can have a dramatic effect on the QoL of many men, as well as their partners. Questionnaire instruments are now available to measure the impact on an individual's QoL [2,7]. However, of equal interest to the physician as the number of patients suffering, is the number presenting and, increasingly, what can be done to identify those non-presenters with ED who have other significant undiagnosed health problems that would benefit from therapy.

7

Increasingly, epidemiologists are trying to assess the magnitude, at least numerically, of the problem and the impact of potential risk factors. Armed with questionnaires such as the Brief Sexual Function Inventory, and the International Index of Erectile Function (IIEF) and its derivatives, we have begun to quantify ED prevalence [7].

A major problem with the assessment of the prevalence is whether the patient in the surgery or community will truthfully disclose the extent of his ED or even want to discuss it at all. In today's post-sildenafil era, many couples will still accept impaired sexual function as being an inevitable consequence of the aging process.

The true prevalence of ED may be masked by men's reticence to discuss their sexual problems

In general, recent surveys have only served to confirm the data of the Massachusetts Male Aging Study (MMAS), 1987–1989 [8]. This community-based survey undertook a random sampling of health status in men between the ages of 40 and 70 years. Although the sampling was confined to the Boston area, more recent surveys have shown that it is probably representative of America's diverse populations, and East and Western Europe. There is no evidence to suggest that the epidemiology of ED is radically different in Latin America, the Pacific Rim, or Japan.

The MMAS shows that over 50% of men in that age range will experience some degree of ED. For almost 80% of these it will be considered mild or moderate (i.e. be potentially manageable in the primary care setting, at least in the first instance). Not surprisingly there is some degree of age relationship; between the fifth and seventh decades the probability of having complete ED triples (Figure 2).

Over 50% of men aged 40–70 years will experience some degree of ED

ED patients are likely to present with many other co-morbidities, particularly hypertension and diabetes, both of which may be controlled or uncontrolled (Figure 3).

Vascular disease of various types has been associated with ED including:

• Myocardial infarction

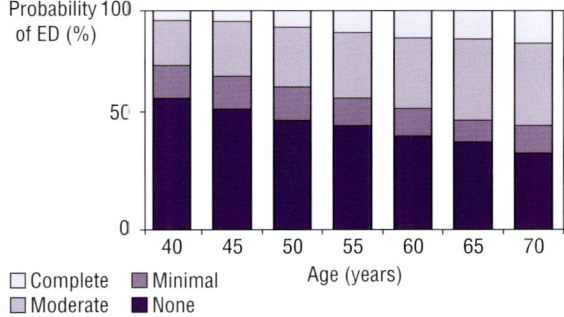

Figure 2.
Probability of ED
relative to age

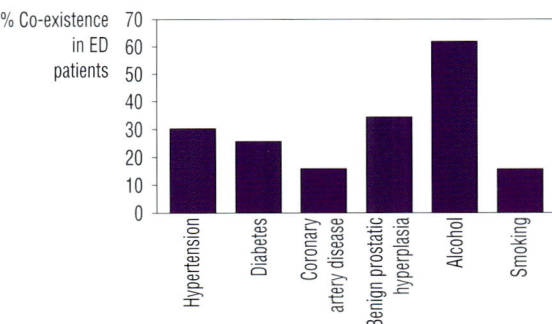

Figure 3. Common
co-morbidities
and associated
risk factors in ED
patients

- Coronary artery disease
- Peripheral vascular disease
- Hypertension and atherosclerosis/dyslipidemia

It has been suggested that ED may often represent the first symptom of atherosclerosis and generalized cardiovascular disease. Its severity might also be considered a marker for the evolution of endothelial dysfunction. This suggestion seems logical, as erectile tissue is a modified vascular bed that will be subject to the full range of pathophysiological changes observed in the general systemic vasculature [6]. Interestingly, there is

9

now evidence that the PDE5 inhibitor drugs used to treat ED may also generally enhance endothelial function [9].

Apart from cardiovascular co-morbidities, other factors increasing the risk of ED are known to include:

- Cigarette smoking
- Alcohol
- Depression
- Several classes of drugs
- Certain surgical procedures (e.g. prostatectomy)
- LUTS

Many of these risk factors are modifiable and help with lifestyle change should form an important part of the treatment plan described later.

Early epidemiological studies conducted in the 1980s and 1990s showed that as few as one in ten patients with ED will present with the problem to their physician. It was anticipated that the general availability of the first effective oral drug, sildenafil, would have a major impact on the management of male sexual health issues. However, even with the arrival of sildenafil and subsequent phosphodiesterase inhibitors, the majority of men still do not seek advice about the condition from their physician [1].

PHYSIOLOGY OF ERECTILE FUNCTION AND DYSFUNCTION

Physiology of normal erectile function [10,11]

Penile erection is the most obvious feature of the male body's response to sexual excitement. It is a complex neurovascular response, influenced by cognitive inputs and facilitated by testosterone [12]. Other features of that response include increases in skin temperature, blood pressure, heart and breathing rates, facial and bodily flushing, dilation of the pupils, and nipple erection. There are also changes in skin's sensitivity to touch. These changes are similar in both men and women.

Erection response to sexual interest is the result of interplay between tactile, visual, auditory, and olfactory signals, combined with cognitive inputs, such as fantasy and memory (Figure 4). These stimuli may be erectogenic or erectolytic, pleasant or unpleasant, and are integrated in specific nuclei within the mid-brain. This balance between stimuli may result

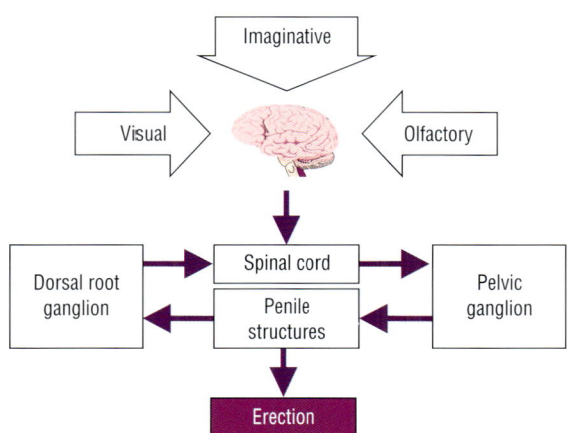

Figure 4. Penile erection is basically a spinal reflex controlled supraspinally, where erectile stimuli can be generated in response to visual, olfactory, and imaginative stimuli

11

in pro-erectile signaling transmitted via the spinal cord, pelvic nerves and cavernous nerves running either side of the prostate gland, before finally terminating around the vascular smooth muscle of the corpora cavernosa.

Erections can also occur in the absence of sexual stimulation. Most men will get spontaneous erections in their sleep, unrelated to sexual thoughts or dreams. Contrary to popular belief, they are not caused by having a full bladder, but probably by unconscious and involuntary changes in the electrical activity of the brain. Men can also get 'reflex' erections, due to activity of sensory–motor linkages within the spinal cord. These are common in men with multiple sclerosis and some types of spinal cord injury.

Cavernosal smooth muscle tone represents an integrated response to many pathways and systems

Erection is a complex series of integrated vascular events culminating in the accumulation of blood under pressure and end-organ rigidity. Fundamentally involved in the intra-penile response are the paired corpus cavernosa that contain the erectile components and are surrounded by a thick fibro-elastic sheath, the tunica albuginea. The erectile tissue comprises multiple interconnecting sinusoidal spaces or lacunae surrounded by trabeculae of smooth muscle (Figure 5).

Figure 5.
Cross-section of
the penis

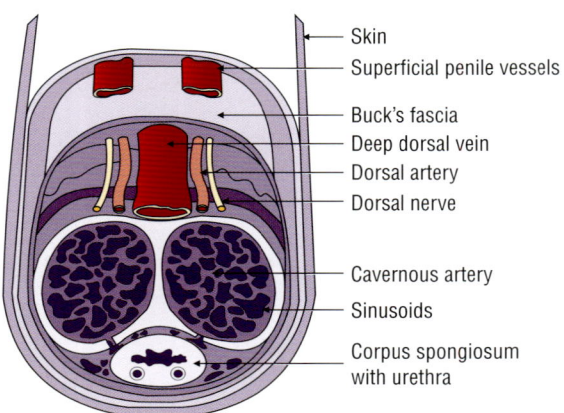

Skin
Superficial penile vessels

Buck's fascia
Deep dorsal vein
Dorsal artery
Dorsal nerve

Cavernous artery

Sinusoids

Corpus spongiosum
with urethra

During erection there is a considerable (up to eightfold) increase in the effective intrapenile blood volume, with corresponding expansion of the trabecular walls and lacunar spaces (Figure 6).

Compression of the plexus of subtunical venules follows, reducing venous outflow. This phenomenon, often referred to as the veno-occlusive mechanism, produces an increase in penile volume (tumescence) and rigidity.

Detumescence occurs through the reversal of this process following contraction of penile smooth muscle. The activation of sympathetic constrictor fibers causes an increase in the tone

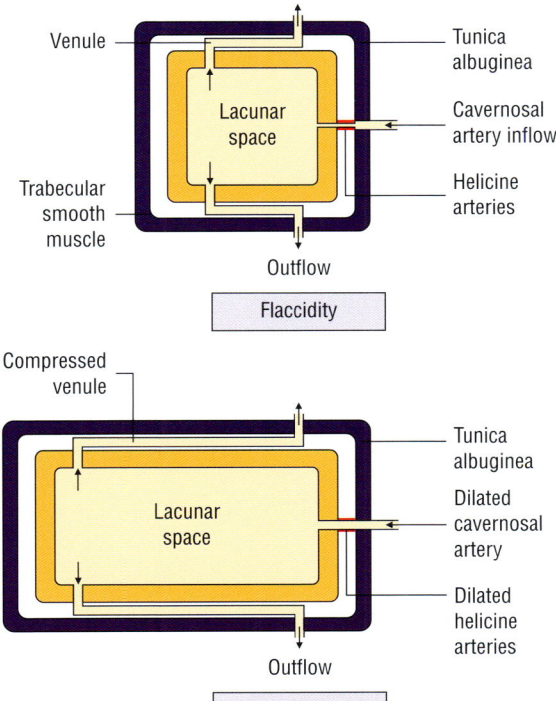

Figure 6. The veno-occlusive mechanism of penile erection

13

of the helicine arteries and the trabeculae. Arterial inflow is reduced and the lacunar space collapses. Decompression of the subtunical venules follows, resulting in increased venous outflow. The penis is returned to the flaccid state.

The overall tone of cavernosal smooth muscle represents an integrated response to many different pathways and systems, the details of which are incompletely understood.

Peripherally, the local balance between contractant and relaxant factors controls the degree of contraction of the smooth muscle and determines the functional status of the penis.

As elsewhere within the autonomic nervous system, sympathetic noradrenergic fibers and parasympathetic cholinergic fibers innervate the cavernosal tissue. In addition, there is innervation from non-adrenergic, non-cholinergic (NANC) nerves.

Within the NANC system a neuromodulator, nitric oxide, is released by nerve endings and endothelial cells, and acts postjunctionally to activate an intracellular enzyme cascade, culminating in erection.

Nitric oxide increases the production of cyclic guanosine monophosphate (cGMP) that decreases intracellular calcium, causing smooth muscle relaxation and penile engorgement (Figure 7). In turn, cGMP is broken down by phosphodiesterases (PDE5). Inhibition of this enzyme forms the basis of the phosphodiesterase inhibitor story.

The central nervous system (CNS) is fundamentally involved in the maintenance of normal erectile and sexual function as it initiates signaling to the penis via the autonomic nervous system and integrates the overall response. An action within the CNS could therefore represent an attractive option as a site of action of an erectogenic drug.

Apomorphine SL was the first example of a centrally active drug approved for use in ED patients; other agents, with a range of target receptors, are being studied. Apomorphine is known to

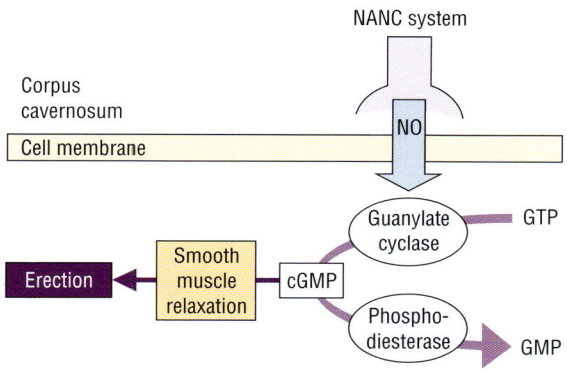

Figure 7. The role of nitric oxide (NO), cyclic guanosine monophosphate (cGMP), and phosphodiesterase type 5 (PDE5) in penile erection

act on dopamine receptors in the brain (Figure 8). A signal is initiated that then travels within the autonomic nervous system to nerves in the pelvic area, dilating the cavernosal vasculature and causing an erection.

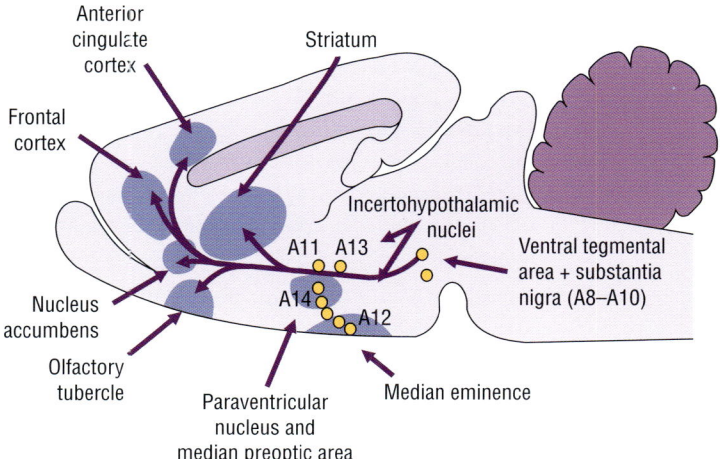

Figure 8. Schematic representation of the involvement of dopaminergic pathways in the control of erectile function in the rat

Pathophysiology

As normal erectile function depends on the delicate balance between vasorelaxation and vasoconstriction of the corporal smooth muscle, disruption of this equilibrium can result in ED. If this critical level of smooth muscle relaxation is not achieved, there will be incomplete resistance to the venous outflow of blood from the corpora and full penile tumescence will be compromised. This is described as veno-occlusive dysfunction and can result from deficiency of the various systems that support the normal integrated response for penile erection.

Vascular factors: Probably the most frequent causes of organic ED are endothelial dysfunction and disturbance of smooth muscle responsiveness within the corporal tissue of the penis.

Decreased arterial flow and perfusion pressure to the lacunar spaces can result from atherosclerosis, or traumatic arterial occlusive disease, of the hypogastric-cavernous arterial bed and may also be a contributory factor.

Excessive outflow through the subtunical venules may result in incomplete tumescence despite sufficient arterial inflow. This can be caused by insufficient relaxation of the trabecular smooth muscle, which may occur in anxious patients with excessive adrenergic-constrictor tone, through damage to the parasympathetic dilator nerves, or by corporal smooth muscle dysfunction.

Neurological factors: Disorders affecting the sacral spinal cord or the peripheral efferent autonomic fibers to the penis can result in incomplete relaxation of the trabecular smooth muscle. Also, disruption of the somatic fibers from the penis that transmit sensory stimuli to the thalamus and sensory cortex (via the pudendal nerve) may also result in ED.

Such neurogenic ED can arise from spinal cord injury, multiple sclerosis, peripheral neuropathies (secondary to diabetes),

Abnormality of the penile blood flow is the most common cause of ED alcoholism, surgical procedures such as radical prostatectomy, or pelvic radiation therapy.

Endocrinological factors: Androgens are necessary for normal sexual development but also influence sexual motivation and behavior. Androgens have been shown to influence the activity of nitric oxide synthase (NOS) and smooth muscle relaxation in the corpus cavernosum. Low levels of bioavailable testosterone may result from a wide range of causes, including changes in the sensitivity of the hypothalamic–pituitary–gonadal axis due to aging, primary hypogonadism, hyperprolactinemia, and the use of leutinizing hormone-releasing hormone (LHRH) agonists.

Diabetes is the most common endocrine abnormality associated as a risk factor for ED. ED may eventually develop in 60% of men with diabetes mellitus. The main causes of the associated ED are thought to arise from the vasculogenic and neurological sequelae of the diabetes. In particular, endothelial and smooth muscle dysfunction and neurological damage to C fibers have been implicated. As many as 40% of diabetic men are also hypogonadal.

More than 50% of diabetic men suffer from associated ED

ED is also associated with hyperthyroidism.

Psychogenic factors: The brain is the most important source of pro-erectile signaling in response to sexual stimulation. Unpleasant tactile, visual, auditory, and olfactory stimuli will tend to inhibit erection. Unpleasant sexual fantasies, perhaps envisaging embarrassment and rejection due to loss of erection with a partner, and memory of poor past sexual experience or relationship dysfunction, will have a similar effect. If these unpleasant, erectolytic stimuli predominate, there may be inadequate central pro-erectile signaling to provide the degree of sustained cavernosal smooth muscle relaxation required for erection.

Penile factors: Peyronie's disease is associated with ED, although it may coexist with other causal factors [13]. In a recent study, nearly a third of men with untreated Peyronie's disease were found to have ED [14]. Changes in the integrity of the fibroelastic components of the trabeculae may result in reduced compression of the subtunical venules. This may be the result of aging, increased cross-linkage of collagen fibers (induced by non-enzymatic glycosylation and hypoxia), altered collagen synthesis associated with hypercholesterolemia, or by trauma to the penis [15].

ERECTILE DYSFUNCTION – ETIOLOGY AND RISK FACTORS

ED is frequently described by its presumed etiology; for example, 'vasculogenic', 'diabetogenic', and 'psychogenic'. These descriptions can be very misleading and it is better always to think of ED as a health problem with multifactorial etiology. This is illustrated in the following two examples.

ED is often of multifactorial origin

> • *A 50-year-old man who has recently been made redundant and has suddenly started experiencing ED for the first time may well have psychological factors as the predominant cause of his problem. However, he might also have atherosclerosis, related to dyslipidemia and smoking, as an additional contributory factor.*
>
> Assuming that his problem is solely 'psychogenic' will result in a missed opportunity for health promotion and disease prevention.

> • *A 23-year-old man who has suffered a spinal cord injury in a road traffic accident and has subsequently developed paraplegia and ED almost certainly has neural damage as the major cause of his problem.*
>
> However, labeling his problem as 'neurogenic' and simply restoring penile rigidity with drugs or appliances will not address the potentially devastating psychological factors affecting his sexuality and self-image.

There are several causes of ED that frequently co-exist.

Psychosexual causes

Psychogenic: Originally, psychological factors were considered to be the most common cause of ED. However, it is now apparent

Psychogenic factors often occur in association with organic factors

that psychological factors alone account for a minority of cases of ED, particularly in older men. It is far more common for psychological and organic factors to co-exist.

Psychosexual factors exist in every man affected by sexual dysfunction, although the patient might protest that they do not. The ability to achieve erection and fulfil one's sexual role is central to the concept of 'maleness', even in the most self-aware and well-adjusted individual.

If psychosexual factors are not identified and addressed, they may lead to treatment failure

The presence of psychosexual factors should always be considered and sought out because, if they are not addressed, they may lead to ED treatment failure.

Inadequate sexual knowledge: Sex education often focuses on reproductive biology, and the prevention of sexually transmitted infection and unwanted pregnancy. Sexual behavior is not usually addressed in any detail. This has led to the acceptance of many 'sexual myths', which lead men to mistakenly believe that they have ED.

Some sexual myths:

- A man should always be interested in sex
- A man should always be able to get an erection in a sexually exciting situation
- A man should always be able to 'give' his partner a 'good' orgasm
- Good sex always involves having a simultaneous orgasm with your partner
- A man should always be in control during sexual intercourse
- A man should always be able to delay his orgasm during intercourse
- Erection problems are always a sign of cancer or other serious illness

These myths are further propagated by the portrayal of sex in the media. Films often show two young, slim, heterosexual and attractive people having prolonged intercourse, the woman enjoying multiple orgasms with the man confidently in control, until they both collapse with an earth-shattering simultaneous orgasm. Alas, sex is not normally like that. On average, intercourse lasts about 9 minutes (although it may be much briefer) [16], is often enjoyable but rarely tumultuous, and we are not all young, slim and attractive.

Unlike the portrayal of sex by the media, intercourse usually lasts about 9 minutes and is rarely tumultuous

Performance anxiety: Performance anxiety can be a cause of ED at any age. Anxiety, whatever its cause, leads to an increase in catecholamine production and sympathetic vasomotor tone, opposing and, potentially, suppressing erection.

General anxiety related to other life events may cause this problem, but performance anxiety is specifically related to erection and intercourse. Typically, the affected man is able to get an erection in response to sexual thoughts and daydreams, and with masturbation (although often not in the presence of his partner). He will usually continue to experience nocturnal and early morning erections. When with his sexual partner, he will experience anxiety that he will not be able to attain or maintain an erection during intercourse. If this has happened in the past, he will remember the embarrassment that this caused him, particularly if his partner made a critical comment about it. He may be able to get an erection during the early stages of the sexual encounter, only to lose it when he attempts penetration, or even during intercourse. There are effective therapies for this problem, psychological and pharmacological, but some men will deny the problem, or conceal it.

Men with performance anxiety or relationship problems will usually have nocturnal, early morning, and masturbatory erections

Relationship problems: ED may be the presenting feature of general relationship problems that extend beyond just the sexual relationship. Where ED is the consequence of a relationship problem, the affected man will often still have an erection with imaginative, visual or masturbatory stimuli, and will usually continue to experience nocturnal and early morning erections.

21

It is only when he is with his sexual partner that he is not able to attain or maintain an erection adequate for intercourse. Occasionally, men will complain of ED, even though they can still achieve erections rigid enough for intercourse. The real problem might be that his partner will not allow intercourse and having ED or failing to respond to ED treatment might be less damaging to his feeling of self-worth. Taking a careful sexual and relationship history will usually clarify the situation. Relationship counseling and couple therapy are often essential parts of the management program.

Simply providing the man with a means to achieve penile rigidity will not help the couple achieve a satisfactory sexual experience and may put the partner at risk of sexual abuse or violence.

Issues of gender identity may not emerge until later life and may present as a sexual dysfunction or relationship problem

Concerns over sexual orientation and gender identity: Although relatively uncommon, concerns over sexual orientation and gender identity do occasionally present with ED. Gay men, who have been raised in an environment where homosexuality is unacceptable, often for cultural or religious reasons, may decide to abstain from sexual behavior altogether or to adopt an unwanted heterosexual lifestyle. They may experience sexual and relationship problems later in life, when they are no longer able to deny their true sexuality.

Men with gender identity disorders have a firm conviction, usually held since childhood, that they are trapped in a body of the wrong gender (transsexualism), which can cause them varying degrees of distress (gender dysphoria). Some will adapt to their unwanted 'maleness' and lead a 'normal' life, perhaps with some adaptations to reduce their dysphoria. Others suffer profound and disabling gender dysphoria. This is characterized by a total disgust with all aspects of their born gender and an all-encompassing desire to change their bodies, by hormones and sometimes by surgery, to the female gender. Transsexuals have no sexual motivation for their desire for gender change; where this is present, transvestism or fetishistic crossdressing are more likely diagnoses.

These issues will sometimes not emerge until mid-life, after the man has married and had a family, when they may present with sexual dysfunction or relationship problems. Frequently, those affected have tried to conform to society's expectations in earlier life and have thrown themselves into what they perceive as typically male occupations, such as joining the military, to prove to themselves and to their peers that they are 'normal men'. Once they have decided that they can no longer live with their 'maleness', they may seek professional help but, not infrequently, they may obtain illicit supplies of feminizing hormones, with obvious negative effects on their sexual function.

Gender identity disorders are rare, affecting around I in 10,000 men and I in 30,000 women [17]. Their effects are frequently devastating and those affected should be referred to a specialist clinic for assistance. Some, but not all, will progress to gender reassignment treatment. They will usually need lifelong help and support.

Although gender identity disorders only affect 1 in 10,000 men, their effects can be devastating

Male-to-female transsexuals who have achieved personal comfort through gender reassignment often wish to enjoy a sexual relationship. Their sexual orientation is not necessarily affected by gender reassignment. If they were sexually attracted to women prior to treatment, they often remain so and may wish to have relationships with other women. Some will be sexually attracted to men and wish to have intercourse with male partners. The genital component of gender reassignment surgery may include vaginoplasty, allowing penetration during intercourse. Female-to-male transsexuals may also wish to be sexually active: a range of options for sexual expression are open to them, including phalloplasty and penile implant surgery.

The sexual problems of transsexuals are beyond the scope of this book, but it should be clear that it is important not to make assumptions about their sexuality and sexual and relationship aspirations.

Cardiovascular disease

Hypertension, coronary heart disease and ED frequently co-exist.

Around 40% or more of ED patients may have some type of cardiovascular disease (Figure 3). Apart from representing a potential causative factor, the presence of underlying cardio-vascular disease should be taken into consideration in patient management [10].

Hypertension: There is a strong association between hypertension and ED. Around 17% of men with untreated hypertension and 24% of men with treated hypertension have ED. It is not only antihypertensive therapy that causes ED, but hypertension itself. There is little evidence that treating hypertension will improve erectile function, although theoretically, the vascular remodeling and improvements in smooth muscle function might enhance erectile response. Hypertension kills people, through stroke, heart failure, and coronary heart disease. The development of ED can be an obstacle to patient compliance with antihypertensive therapy. Treating ED should not compromise achieving good blood pressure control using contemporary treatment guidelines [1,2]. Most men with well-controlled hypertension can be safely and effectively treated for ED; uncontrolled hypertension should be brought under control before ED therapy is initiated [18].

Men on such treatment should be routinely asked about their sexual and erectile function, regardless of age. There is no good evidence that changing antihypertensive agents improves erectile function. Unless there is a strong temporal relationship between the introduction of a new drug and the onset of ED, it is unlikely that withdrawing a drug will be of benefit.

There are theoretical grounds for suggesting that alpha-blockers, such as doxazosin, are less likely to cause ED than other agents. However, there is a potential interaction between alpha-blockers and PDE5 inhibitors that may result in significant hypotension in some patients. Caution should be exercised before co-prescribing these drugs, making reference to manufacturers' recommendations. Angiotensin-converting enzyme (ACE) inhibitors, angiotensin II (ATII) type I receptor blockers, and calcium channel blockers seem to have a fairly neutral effect on erections (Figure 9) [19,20].

Modern beta-blockers, particularly atenolol, are often blamed for causing ED, although the evidence for this is relatively poor. Propranolol and the older, centrally acting antihypertensives (e.g. clonidine) are more likely to cause ED. The evidence for thiazide diuretics causing ED is mixed but several long-term studies show a negative impact on erectile function [21].

Coronary heart disease: Coronary heart disease is associated with many of the same risk factors as ED, including dyslipidemia, hypertension, diabetes, smoking, and sedentary lifestyle. Arterial disease in the heart is just one site in a generalized arteriopathy, which is likely to affect the ileal, pelvic, pudendal,

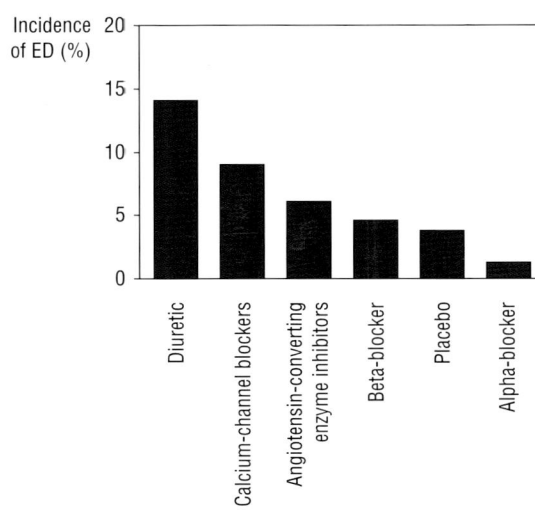

Figure 9. Incidence of ED among men receiving antihypertensive medications

and penile arteries, too. Urologists have been known to refer to ED as 'atherosclerosis of the penis' [6].

Research has shown that 44% of men who have had a myocardial infarction also have ED. This is probably due to more generalized vascular disease, rather than impaired cardiac function. Psychosexual issues may also affect erection in men with coronary heart disease. They, and their partners, may be afraid that the exertion and excitement of intercourse could precipitate a further coronary episode.

The vast majority of men with coronary heart disease can safely resume sexual activity and use ED therapies. Education and appropriate counseling about sex should be given to all men with coronary heart disease so that the majority can continue to enjoy this important aspect of their relationship [6].

Men with unstable heart disease, a history of recent myocardial infarction, poorly compensated heart failure or unstable dysrhythmia are exceptions. Men taking nitric oxide-donor drugs must not take PDE5 inhibitors because of associated hypotension. ACE inhibitors, modern beta-blockers and calcium channel blockers, in normal doses, are unlikely to be a major contributory factor to the development of ED. Much the same can be said of nitrates and nicorandil. However, their use will absolutely preclude the use of PDE5 inhibitors as an ED treatment option. Unlike ACE inhibitors and beta-blockers, they convey no prognostic benefit with regard to the development of further coronary episodes. As such, one can consider their replacement with other anti-anginal agents [22].

Not all men carrying glyceryl trinitrate tablets or spray will be suffering from angina

Some men may have been given a supply of glyceryl trinitrate tablets or spray upon their discharge from hospital following a coronary event, even though they do not have angina. They will often have been told to carry it with them at all times and will have dutifully obeyed these instructions for many years, regularly refilling their prescription from their family physician, even though they never use the drug. Men who never use this medication should be reviewed by their cardiologist or family physician and, if appropriate, be advised that they do not need to carry nitrate therapy, thus enabling them to have PDE5 inhibitors as an ED treatment option.

Diabetics can be difficult to treat as their response rate to drug therapies may be lower

Endocrine disorders

Endocrine disorders may cause ED and, in some cases, may be one of the few etiologies whose resolution might lead to a 'cure'. Consequently, such disorders should be routinely sought out in the assessment of men with ED. However, as ED is multifactorial in origin, an endocrine disorder might be only a contributory factor to the problem. Endocrine disorders commonly seen in ED patients include diabetes, thyroid disease, androgen deficiency, and hyperprolactinemia.

Diabetes: Diabetes is the most common endocrine abnormality associated as a risk factor for ED (Figure 10).

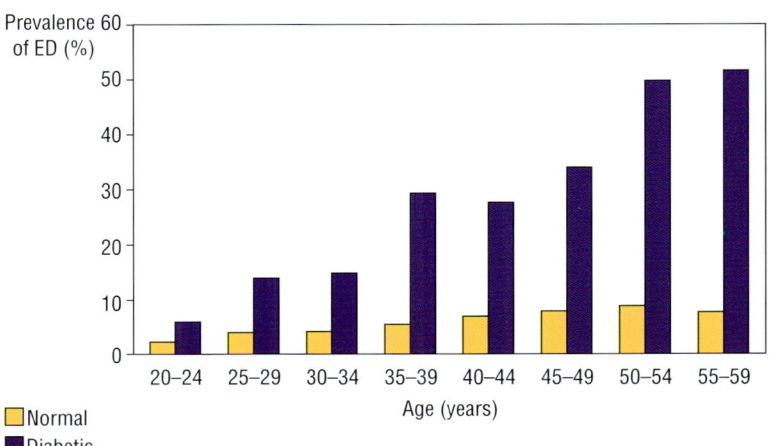

Figure 10. Prevalence of ED in diabetic men compared to 'normal men'

The prevalence of ED is almost three times higher in diabetic men (28%) than in the non-diabetic population (9.6%) [23]. Diabetes is associated with dyslipidemia, neuropathy and smooth muscle dysfunction, all of which are associated with ED. Although there is little evidence that improving glycemic control in diabetics improves their erectile function, there is some evidence that high glycosylated hemoglobin (HbA1C) levels impair smooth muscle function. Thus, there are theoretical grounds for believing that improved diabetic control is advantageous in ED, although this alone will not normally restore erections. Diabetics are a difficult group to treat for ED, as their response rate to drug therapies, such as sildenafil, is lower than in most other groups. Diabetic men also commonly have reduced androgen levels.

Thyroid disease: There is an association between hyperthyroidism and ED. This may be due to a hyperthyroidism-related increase in sex hormone-binding globulin (SHBG) levels and increased aromatization of testosterone to estrogen [24]. Restoring the euthyroid state may resolve the ED.

Androgen deficiency: Androgen deficiency in the adult male becomes more common with increasing age [24], but its management remains controversial. As well as sexual dysfunction, androgen deficiency is associated with osteoporosis, dyslipidemia, metabolic syndrome and depression. Far from being a benign consequence of aging, it is a significant cause of increased cardiovascular risk. Androgens act at several sites in the sexual response system: within the CNS, peripheral nitrergic nerves, and corpora cavernosa. Androgen deficiency may affect sexual interest, erections, and responsiveness to PDE5 inhibitors [12].

Identification of androgen deficiency is based upon the identification of its non-specific clinical features and blood testing. Choice of assay is between total, free (unbound to plasma proteins), and bioavailable testosterone (unbound to SHBG). Free testosterone is probably the most reliable assay, as it is not affected by changes in SHBG levels. However, the most reliable direct measure, equilibrium dialysis, is only available in research laboratories; commercial radioimmunoassay are frequently unreliable [25]. Calculated free testosterone is probably the best available surrogate [26]. It can be derived from total testosterone, SHBG and albumin levels; an on-line calculator can be found at *www.issam.ch*.

As there is a diurnal variation in testosterone release, samples for testosterone assay should be drawn in the morning, between 08.00 and 11.00. The assay should be repeated after 2 or 3 weeks, as testosterone is released in a pulsatile manner, as well as with diurnal variation, and the result of a single assay may be misleading.

Men with symptoms of androgen deficiency should be assessed and androgen replacement given on its merits [27]. A screening questionnaire for androgen-deficiency symptoms has been published, although it is of low specificity [28].

There is no evidence that giving testosterone to men with ED and normal androgen levels restores or improves their erectile function. Testosterone should be prescribed under specialist supervision for men with established hypogonadism. Prior assessment and safety monitoring should be performed according to contemporary authoritative guidelines [24].

Hyperprolactinemia: Hyperprolactinemia is associated with ED, loss of sexual interest and anorgasmia [29]. It is frequently accompanied by androgen deficiency, as high prolactin levels suppress LH production and, consequently, cause hypogonadism.

Hyperprolactinemia should be excluded by blood testing in all men with reduced sexual interest. Moderate elevation of prolactin levels (<1000 mIU/l) is unlikely to cause ED.

Hyperprolactinemia is often due to stress and drugs (notably metoclopramide, chlorpromazine, and several other antipsychotics). Only about one in ten of these men will be found to have a prolactin-secreting pituitary tumor, but these must not

Hyperprolactinemia should be excluded in all men with reduced sexual drive

Prolactin-secreting tumors may only be found in 1 in 10 men with hyperprolactinemia, but must not be missed be missed. Hyperprolactinemia is common in men on dialysis for chronic renal failure. Unless an obvious cause is found and the prolactin levels return to normal, referral to an endocrinologist is advisable.

Neurological disorders

Several neurological disorders may contribute to ED in some patients and should be considered in relation to treatment options. These include stroke, epilepsy, spinal cord injury, multiple sclerosis, and Parkinson's disease [21].

Stroke: Men who have had strokes are more likely to have ED. This is as likely to be due to generalized arteriopathy or be a consequence of physical disability, rather than the brain injury itself. If self-image or cognitive functions are impaired, there may be a secondary effect on erection. The centers in the brain controlling sexual response are mainly located in the mid-brain and intimately related to vital structures, such as the vasomotor center. A brain injury specifically affecting these centers is likely to be fatal.

Provided that the neurological and cardiovascular problems are stable, most men with ED following a stroke can be treated safely and effectively.

Epilepsy: Epilepsy is associated with reduced sexual drive. This is due to the neurological disorder itself, rather than the drugs used to treat it. Several analeptic drugs have been implicated as causes of ED and anorgasmia. Some of the newer analeptic agents are said to be less likely to cause sexual dysfunctions. Most men with epilepsy can be treated for ED safely and effectively.

Spinal cord injury: The level and severity of the spinal cord injury will determine the degree and type of ED experienced. Many men will still have reflexogenic erections, which are transient and poorly sustained, in response to genital stimulation, but lose the ability to achieve central erections in response to cognitive sexual excitement. Reflexogenic erections can be particularly frustrating, as they will often occur at inappropriate times or detumesce during intercourse.

Men with spinal cord injuries require careful assessment and follow-up, as there may be a variety of associated problems, such as:

- Anorgasmia and anejaculation (often but not always)
- Problems of physical disability
- Continence problems
- Changes in self-image
- Relationship issues
- Fertility concerns

Most men with spinal cord injury can be treated safely and effectively for ED. Men with high lesions, at or above D4, should be treated with care, because of the risk of provoking a hypertensive crisis due to autonomic dysreflexia during intercourse.

Multiple sclerosis: Multiple sclerosis is strongly associated with ED and it is occasionally the presenting symptom of this troublesome disorder. Most men with multiple sclerosis can be treated for ED safely and effectively.

Parkinson's disease and multi-system atrophy: Men with multi-system atrophy and Parkinson's disease are more likely to experience sexual dysfunction and ED. The reasons for this are complex and incompletely understood. Changes in self-image, physical disability, depression, and cognitive impairment all play a part, but there may be more specific causes. In Parkinson's disease there is a degeneration of the dopaminergic neurons of the nigrostriatal tract. It is possible that a similar degenerative process affects the dopaminergic neurons in the hypothalamus and mid-brain that are involved in central mediation of sexual response, which are closely related anatomically to the nigrostriatal tract. Most men with Parkinson's disease and multi-system atrophy can be treated safely and effectively for ED, although general impairment of sexual function will increase as the disorders progress.

Mental health problems

Depression: Depression and its treatments are strongly associated with ED and other sexual dysfunctions [30]. Sometimes depression causes these problems and sometimes the problems cause depression. Taking a careful history may help clarify the situation. Both problems warrant treatment and should be managed concurrently. There is evidence that treating ED can improve depressive symptoms [31]. However, depression is a serious, potentially life-threatening condition and should be treated aggressively.

All antidepressants have the potential to cause sexual dysfunction. Modern tricyclic antidepressants (TCAs) are probably no worse than selective serotonin reuptake inhibitors (SSRIs) in this respect. Older TCAs, with marked sedative and anticholinergic effects, are more likely to cause ED. SSRIs are known to delay orgasm or even cause anorgasmia. They are sometimes used as a treatment for premature ejaculation. They can also cause loss of sexual drive and, less frequently, ED. Newer antidepressant agents, particularly those not working through the serotonin system (e.g. mirtazepine, nefazodone, and reboxetine) may be less prone to cause sexual side effects.

Patients who are depressed or who are receiving treatment for depression should be routinely questioned about sexual function while reviewing the management of their depressive illness. For some, sexual intimacy allows them to escape from the pain of their depressive illness. It is both appropriate and a kindness to offer treatment for ED to affected men with depression.

Depression is strongly associated with loss of sex drive, ED and orgasmic dysfunction

All antidepressants have the potential to cause sexual dysfunction

Most antipsychotics cause hyper-prolactinemia, which can in turn result in loss of sex drive and ED

Schizophrenia and other psychoses: Sexual function in men with schizophrenia and other psychotic illness is often neglected while attention is paid to their mental health problems.

Most men with relapsing psychotic disorders remain well for most of the time and wish to enjoy sexual relationships. The majority of antipsychotic agents, including several atypical antipsychotics, are centrally acting dopamine antagonists and cause hyperprolactinemia. This can, in turn, cause loss of sexual drive and ED.

The atypical antipsychotic quetiapine seems less prone to cause sexual side effects. Anticholinergics, used to ameliorate other side effects, can add to the problem. Modification of dosage or drug can improve sexual function, but this should only be attempted in collaboration with a psychiatrist.

Men with schizophrenia and other psychotic illness should be routinely asked about sexual function and, where appropriate, treatment should be offered.

Cognitive impairment and dementia: The development of cognitive impairment and dementia often has a devastating effect on a relationship. However, some couples continue to enjoy a satisfactory sexual relationship and, provided that the rights of the cognitively impaired partner are respected and protected, treatment for ED should be offered.

Urological problems

Benign prostatic hyperplasia: Benign prostatic hyperplasia (BPH) is a common condition in the aging male and is associated with a range of sexual dysfunctions. In one study, over 44% of men with severe LUTS complained of unsuccessful coitus, compared with only 13% of those with milder symptoms. However, a direct causal relationship between BPH, LUTS and ED seems unlikely [32]. Loss of sexual drive, orgasmic and ejaculatory problems have been reported in untreated BPH, as well as ED [19].

BPH is common in the aging male and a significant number of men with LUTS complain of unsuccessful coitus

33

Treatments for BPH are also associated with ED and sexual dysfunction. Ejaculatory problems are the most common, with both medical and surgical treatment. According to one meta-analysis, the incidence of ED following transurethral resection of the prostate (TURP) is between 3% and 32%. However, a more recent prospective study suggested that TURP does not cause ED [19].

ED is associated with many of the BPH treatments

Psychological factors, including the man's response to ejaculatory dysfunction, may play an important part.

There is evidence that the 5-α-reductase inhibitor finasteride results in a reduction in libido in roughly 5% of BPH patients and a reduction in erectile functioning (Figure 11). In general, alpha-blockers have little effect on sexual function, although tamsulosin has been shown to produce retrograde ejaculation in up to 15% of BPH patients.

To date, all potentially curative treatments for prostate cancer cause ED in a high proportion of men

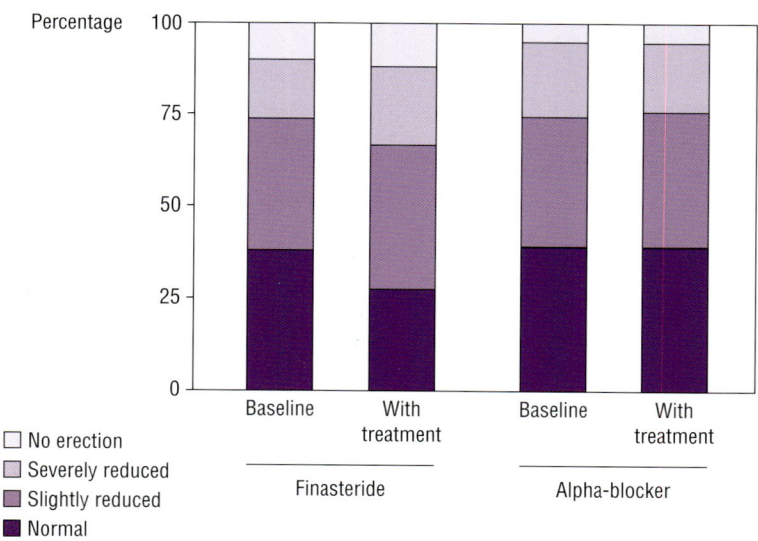

Figure 11. Effect of finasteride on erectile function compared to an alpha-blocker

Most men with BPH, or on BPH treatment, can be safely and effectively treated for ED.

Prostate cancer: It is very unusual for ED to be the first symptom of prostate cancer, although many men with ED are very concerned that it might be in their case. It is often treatments for prostate cancer that lead to sexual dysfunction, rather than the disease itself.

Medical treatments to suppress androgen action, such as GnRH agonists (goserelin, leuprorelin) or androgen receptor blockers (cyproterone acetate, flutamide, bicalutamide), frequently cause a marked loss of sexual interest and ED [21]. This effect is most pronounced with GnRH analogs and can last for many months after treatment is withdrawn; it seems to be less of a problem with the androgen receptor blocker bicalutamide. Even so, around 50% of men taking bicalutamide 50 mg daily will have ED [33].

ED is a common problem following radical prostatectomy. Studies have reported ED rates of 30–100% following such surgery. The problem usually develops immediately following surgery; suggested mechanisms for this are intraoperative injury to the cavernous nerves and/or arteries, and structural alterations to the corpora cavernosal that are disruptive of the veno-occlusive mechanism [34]. Nerve-sparing procedures may reduce the risk of post-operative ED. Radical radiotherapy is also associated with ED in about 40% of men, although the onset is often delayed for 6–18 months. Brachytherapy, where small seeds of radioactive material are implanted into the prostate, is associated with ED in about 50% of men. It seems that all currently available [35], potentially curative treatments for prostate cancer cause ED in a significant proportion of men.

Radical prostatectomy is strongly associated with ED, with an incidence of 30–100% reported in different series. Research suggests that pre-operative erectile function status, age and intra-operative nerve sparing are the main determinants of post-operative potency [36]. There is evidence that early introduction of pharmacotherapy to restore erections at an early stage may result in better recovery rates [34].

Most men with prostate cancer can be safely treated for ED, although those who have undergone radical surgery or radiotherapy have lower response rates to treatment.

Other surgery: About 30% of men will develop ED following radical surgery for rectal cancer, although this may be improved with nerve-sparing surgery; retrograde ejaculation is also observed [37]. Other surgical procedures associated with ED include cystectomy, and aortic and femoral grafting.

Peyronie's disease and other penile disorders: Peyronie's disease is a disorder affecting the penis, characterized by penile pain, a lump within the penile shaft, and abnormal angulation of the erect penis. Sometimes, all three features are not present. It is thought to affect 3% of men, although it is probably under-reported to doctors. However, Peyronie's disease is identified in about 16% of men presenting with ED to a specialist clinic [38].

In Peyronie's disease fibrous plaques in the tunica albuginea result in characteristic penile curvature on erection

In Peyronie's disease, palpable fibrous plaques appear within the tunica albuginea. When the penis becomes erect, it inflates unevenly and tends to bend around the plaque, causing the characteristic, deformed appearance.

It is possible that the deformity of the tunica albuginea disrupts the normal veno-occlusive mechanism essential to erection, leading to the development of ED. More often, the penis tends to bend and buckle around the fibrous plaque, whilst the proximal and distal segments of the penis remain erect. This can render intercourse just as impossible as ED. Finally, many men are severely embarrassed by the appearance of their penis. They may also be distressed by pain on erection, which might last for several months. This adds a further, psychogenic component to their ED.

Men with Peyronie's disease may experience pain and associated psychogenic ED, in addition to penile deformity

Most men with Peyronie's disease can be safely treated for ED. However, the effectiveness of treatment will depend upon the severity of the deformity. If the penis is too bent to facilitate penetration, specific treatment to correct the deformity will be necessary. However, surgical treatment for Peyronie's disease may also result in ED [39].

Other penile problems, such as infective balanitis, balanitis xerotica obliterans, phimosis and STD may also affect sexual function. They should be sought out and treated on their own merits.

Trauma: Direct injury to the penis, blunt as well as sharp, may disrupt the tunica albuginea and corpora cavernosa, causing penile fracture and, possibly, penile deformity and ED. Penile neurovascular injury may also occur. These problems are more likely in injuries resulting in urethral rupture. Occasionally, a blow to the penis will result in an arterio-venous fistula. This may present as ED, or as 'high-flow' priapism. The erection of 'high-flow' priapism is not usually painful or completely rigid; it is characterized by a persistent warm tumescence. The more common 'low-flow' priapism, which may result from injection of pharmacological agents or sickle cell disease, is usually cold, rigid, dusky, and painful. It constitutes a urological emergency, as delay in treatment may lead to permanent damage to corpora and intractable ED.

Pelvic fractures, commonly seen following road traffic accidents, or straddle injuries, may cause vascular and nerve damage and, consequently, ED. Less severe trauma, such as pressure from a bicycle saddle on neurovascular structures, has also been suggested as a cause of ED [40].

'Lifestyle' and iatrogenic causes

'Lifestyle' and ED: As might be expected, smoking, sedentary lifestyle and obesity are associated with ED. It is obviously good practice to encourage men with ED to stop smoking, drink less alcohol, take more exercise, and lose weight. This may reduce their risk of developing cardiovascular and other lifestyle-related diseases, but, apart from taking more exercise, there is no objective evidence that it will improve their erectile function. Increased physical activity, if begun by mid-life, may reduce the burden of ED in older men [41].

Drugs: A wide variety of drugs have been blamed for causing ED or other sexual dysfunction [21], frequently on the basis of single case reports and anecdote. The evidence for a causal relationship between many cardiovascular drugs and ED is poor. Psychoactive drugs may cause sexual dysfunction through general sedation, hormonal effects (several antipsychotics cause hyperprolactinemia), or activity at neuroreceptor sites involved in the mediation of sexual response. The following lists some of the drugs that have been implicated:

Diuretics	*Thiazides*
	Spironolactone
Antihypertensives	*Methyldopa*
	Clonidine
	Reserpine
	Beta-blockers
	Guanethidine
	Verapamil
Cardiac/circulatory	*Clofibrate*
	Gemfibrozil
	Digoxin
Tranquillisers	*Phenothiazines*
	Butyrophenones
Antidepressants	*TCAs*
	MAOIs
	Lithium
	SSRIs
H2 antagonists	*Cimetidine*
	Ranitidine

Hormones	Estrogens/progesterone
	Corticosteroids
	Cyproterone acetate
	5-α-reductase inhibitors
	LHRH agonists
Cytotoxic agents	Cyclophosphamide
	Methotrexate
	Roferon-A
Anticholinergics	Disopyramide
	Anticonvulsants

ASSESSMENT OF ERECTILE DYSFUNCTION

General principles

The purpose of clinical assessment is to identify and agree the nature of the individual's/couple's problem(s), why it has occurred, their aims for treatment outcome, and whether this may realistically be achieved with biomedical or pysychotherapeutic interventions. These are summarized in Figure 12.

The 'diagnosis' of the causes of a complex, multifactorial problem requires a holistic approach, considering biomedical, psychological, behavioral, partner, and relationship issues.

A list of predisposing, precipitating and maintaining factors is given below.

Figure 12.
Principles
for clinical
assessment of
patients with ED

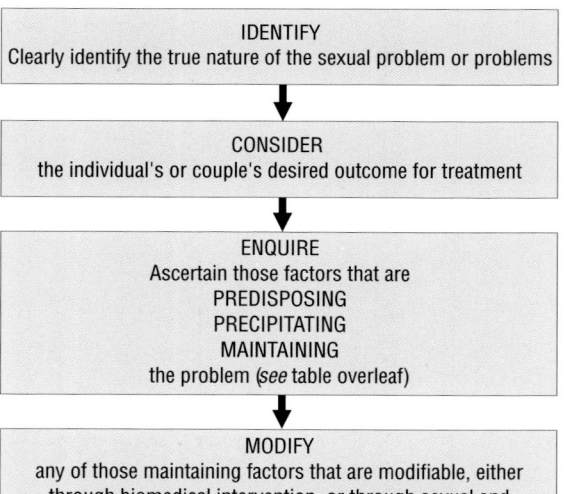

Working with individuals and with couples

When assessing a sexual problem, it is almost always desirable to see both partners in a sexual relationship, even if there only seems to be one person affected. The partner can provide important additional information and may also need help with their own sexual problems. Co-existing problems in both partners are common, and may be an obstacle to successful treatment [42].

Co-existence of problems in both partners is common and an obstacle to successful treatment

Predisposing	Precipitating	Maintaining
Lack of sexual knowledge	New relationship	Relationship problems
Poor past sexual experience	Acute relationship problems	Poor communication between partners
Relationship problems	Family or social pressures	Lack of knowledge about treatment options
Religious or cultural beliefs	Pregnancy and childbirth	Ongoing physical or mental health problems
Restrictive upbringing	Other major life events	Other sexual problems in the man or his partner
Unclear sexual or gender preference	Partner's menopause	Drugs
Previous sexual abuse	Acute physical or mental health problems	
Physical or mental health problems	Lack of knowledge about normal changes of aging	
Other sexual problems in the man or his partner	Other sexual problems in the man or his partner	
Drugs	Drugs	

41

Sexual dysfunctions in women are a common problem, affecting perhaps 40% of women, although only around 20% have sought help. Problems with desire, genital and subjective arousal, orgasm, and sexual pain have been described. Their assessment and management is beyond the scope of this book. However, these problems are important: they can cause significant distress, may have a negative impact upon ED treatment outcome, and, importantly, are amenable to treatment. Women with concerns over sexual function may benefit from a holistic biomedical and psychosexual evaluation, and should be strongly encouraged to seek professional help.

Post-menopausal women who are partners of men with ED and who have not had intercourse for some time may notice impaired vaginal lubrication and elasticity. This is often due to estrogen deficiency-related atrophic vaginitis. They should be warned that this might occur and be made aware that they should seek treatment if necessary. This advice should be given concurrently with any ED treatment, rather than waiting for the problem to emerge.

In practice, many men are reluctant to involve their partners and, not infrequently, the partner does not wish to attend. There are frequently perfectly valid reasons for this but, occasionally, the absence of a partner may indicate that they are unwilling to allow resumption of sexual intercourse. It is very important to ask men attending alone about their general relationship satisfaction and to solicit information about their view of their partner's perception of their problem.

Sometimes, men with ED will admit that they have not told their partner that they are seeking treatment and suggest that they 'want it to be a surprise' for them. This may well be the case for a partner who has not had intercourse for several years and is suddenly confronted with an unwelcome erect penis. While it might not be appropriate to insist that a man tells his partner that he is seeking ED treatment, he should be strongly encouraged to do so.

Principles of taking a sexual history

Taking a sexual history presents different challenges to the physician, not least because most physicians have had little or no training or experience in doing so. Many people, both lay and professional, find talking about sex uncomfortable to a greater or lesser degree. Many people, again both lay and professional, have their own beliefs, rooted in the culture and religion of their upbringing, about what is acceptable sexual behavior and what is not. The ability to talk freely about sexual behavior and lifestyles is a skill that must be acquired if the physician is to help people with sexual problems. If, for whatever reason, they find themselves unable to do this, it is better that they acknowledge the fact and promptly refer people with sexual problems to a colleague. There is no shame in doing this, but it is shameful to withhold treatment or discriminate against people who adopt sexual lifestyles and behaviors that are legally acceptable, but at variance with our own belief system [43].

In general, the following principles of taking a sexual history should be considered.

- Use appropriate language – for the understanding and comfort of the couple. Keep checking that you all agree what particular words and expressions mean. For example, 'arousal' may mean 'sexual excitement' to one person, 'erection' to another and 'orgasm' to a third.

- Allow adequate time for the consultation. Even relatively straightforward problems will take 20–30 minutes to assess. This may seem like a long time, but is really not much different from the time that is spent in assessing a patient with newly diagnosed asthma or diabetes. It may not be possible to accommodate a consultation of that length in a normal clinic appointment. In this case, a special appointment or, less desirably, spreading the assessment over more than one consultation might be more appropriate.

Most physicians have little or no training experience of taking a sexual history

- Privacy and confidentiality – ensure that complete privacy is possible and that the confidentiality of both partners is maintained.

- Consider the cultural and religious beliefs of the couple and how these might affect their sexual behavior, their response to questions of an intimate nature, and the acceptability of physical examination to them.

- Beware of recording third-party information in the patient's notes. You should not record identifiable details of the partner's sexual behavior or problems other than in their own notes.

Guidelines for taking a sexual history

Be sure to elicit the following information:

Do you think that your sex drive (libido, interest in sex) is normal?

1. How frequently do you feel the need to have sex?

2. Do you occasionally experience spontaneous sexual thoughts, daydreams or fantasies?

What is the exact nature of the problem?

> *This is vital, so that you can be sure that it is ED that is the problem and not premature ejaculation or a relationship problem.*

1. Ask the patient to describe exactly what happens when he anticipates lovemaking, right from the beginning.

> *This may reveal a different problem or the couple's poor sexual knowledge.*

2. How does it affect you and your partner's (if you have one) relationship?

> *ED may be the cause or consequence of a relationship problem, and sometimes it's both.*

3. Is it important to you both?

    If it is not important, ask why he has attended – perhaps he is worried that he might have cancer.

4. Can you get a good quality erection sometimes with masturbation or in other erotic situations.

    The ability to get erections at some times and not others – 'situational' ED – makes it unlikely that physical factors are the major cause of the problem.

5. Do you get erections at other times, even if only briefly, at night or upon wakening?

    Again, 'situational' ED is unlikely to have a primarily organic cause, whereas 'global' ED may well be organic.

How long have you had the problem?

1. When did you first decide that you had a problem?

2. Did it start suddenly or gradually?

    Sudden onset, unless related to an injury, illness or medical intervention, suggests a predominantly psychosexual etiology.

3. When were you and your partner last able to enjoy satisfactory lovemaking together?

4   Does the problem occur every time you try to make love?

    Intermittent ED is strongly suggestive of a predominantly psychosexual etiology, persistent ED is more likely to be organic.

What is your partner's attitude toward this problem?

    This information is essential but is more reliably assessed if the partner is willing and able to attend the assessment as well.

What do you think is causing the problem?

    Some couples are convinced that their sexual problems are related to a serious and, as yet, undiagnosed medical problem. Occasionally they are correct, but even if they are not, their concerns should be addressed and alleviated.

1. Do you think there is something the matter with you?

2. Do you think there is something the matter with your partner?

What would you and your partner like to achieve as a result of treatment?

> *The obvious answer is 'to be able to have sexual intercourse again', but this is not always the case. Couples have sex for a variety of reasons, usually for recreation and to maintain intimacy, but also for reproduction, assertion of role, relief from pain, or even to exert power and control. Understanding the couple's sexual goals is of considerable help when planning treatment, particularly if those goals are unachievable or incompatible.*

Examination

The routine assessment examination of a man with ED is straightforward and should only take a few minutes to carefully perform. Some authorities include digital rectal examination of the prostate gland.

1. Assess the general appearance and affect

   Are there signs of other illness, such as depression, thyroid disease or Parkinson's disease?

   Is there evidence of physical disability?

2. Assess the secondary sexual characteristics

   Is the distribution and quality of facial, body, and pubic hair normal? Is there normal muscle development?

   Is the body fat distribution 'android' or 'gynecoid'?

3. Inspect and palpate the penile shaft, then examine and, if possible, retract and replace the foreskin

   Are there any lumps or tender areas in the flaccid penis, suggesting Peyronie's disease?

Are the foreskin and glans penis healthy?

Does retraction cause pain?

Is there evidence of balanitis, warts or other STD?

4. Inspect and palpate the scrotal contents

Are the testes of normal size and consistency? (Men with small, atrophic testes are not necessarily androgen deficient.)

5. Check the blood pressure in accordance with contemporary guidelines

Investigations

The following should be performed for all men with ED. It should be recalled that ED and cardiovascular disease share identical risk factors; all men with ED should have a thorough cardiovascular risk assessment.

1. Fasting glucose

2. Urinalysis for glucose

This a poor screening test for diabetes but, if blood sampling is impossible, it is better than nothing. Much the same can be said of stick testing for blood glucose

3. Total, HDL and cholesterol, and triglycerides

ED and atherosclerosis share common risk factors; men with ED should always be assessed for dyslipidemia

4. Total testosterone, SHBG, and albumen

Calculated free testosterone (FT) is the best readily-available assessment of androgen status; these results can be used to calculate FT. Morning testing is recommended

5. Prolactin

Consider also checking:

1. Thyroid function

2. Prostate-specific antigen (PSA)

Routine PSA screening in men with ED is recommended by some authorities, but practice varies from country to country.

Special investigations: Special investigations are rarely necessary and only indicated if a man fails to respond as expected to medical therapy, or if it is suspected that his ED is due to a congenital or acquired vascular malformation. In such cases, the man should be referred to an appropriate secondary care specialist interested in sexual function problems. This will normally be a urologist, although not all urologists have an interest in ED or penile vascular surgery.

Diagnosing, summarizing, and explaining the problem

Having completed the assessment, the physician should have a list of predisposing, precipitating, and maintaining factors that have contributed to the problem. For example, a 50-year-old hypertensive man comes to the surgery complaining that he is unable to get an erection. His assessment reveals the following information.

Predisposing	Precipitating	Maintaining
Sexually restrictive upbringing	New sexual relationship	Performance anxiety
Poor sexual knowledge		Unable to discuss sexual problems with his partner
Poor past sexual experience in an unhappy marriage		Away from home during week on business travel
Highly stressful occupation		Hypertension
Away from home during week on business travel		Treatment with ACE inhibitor
Hypertension		Perimenopausal partner with symptoms of atrophic vaginitis
Treatment with ACE inhibitor		

It would be inadequate to simply blame the ED on his hypertension, and to either change his medication or to just offer him a drug or appliance.

He, and preferably his partner as well, need an explanation of why the problem has occurred, what is keeping it going, and what might be done to resolve it. He may well need some simple sex education, so that he has a better understanding of his sexual response and how aging, performance anxiety, and his partner can affect it.

Being away at work all week and having to 'perform' at weekends cannot be helping this. He may need help and encouragement to talk to her about the sexual aspects of their relationship. She may also need information and education about her own sexuality and also about options for dealing with menopausal symptoms.

With this in mind, the treatment package includes individual or couple education, simple psychosexual therapy aimed at improving the couple's understanding of sexuality and reducing his performance anxiety, and possibly biomedical interventions for both partners.

Who to refer? While the non-ED specialist physician can manage the majority of men with ED successfully, the following groups might be referred to a specialist ED service:

- Men who require treatment or services not provided within the practice (e.g. a full sexual and relationship therapy service, or intracavernosal injections)

- Men who fail to respond to treatment as expected

- Men with sexual problems, behaviors or lifestyles that interfere with the physician's ability to deal with them in an open and non-judgmental manner

- Men with sexual problems related to essential psychotropic or other medication, who do not respond to therapies offered within the practice

- Men who have developed ED following a pelvic or genital injury

TREATMENT PLANNING

The overall approach is summarized in Figure 13.

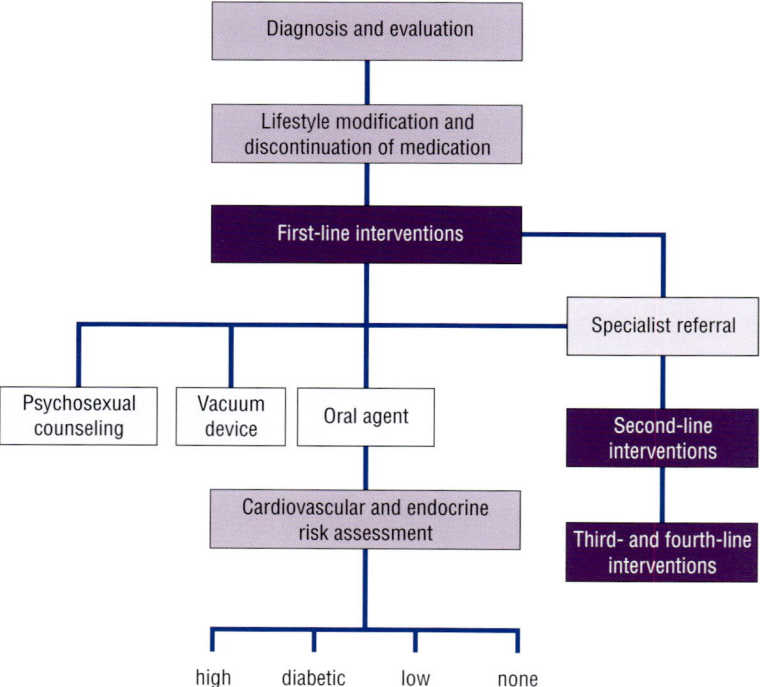

Figure 13. Treatment algorithm for the management of ED patients

The treatment plan should always include the following components.

Education: Provide adequate information for the man, and preferably his partner, to understand why he has ED and how his problem compares with the general population. Many

First-line therapies

Basic sex education, information-giving and simple behavioral advice

Oral therapies: 'as required'

- Sildenafil
- Tadalafil
- Vardenafil
- Apomorphine SL

Vacuum erection devices

Sexual and relationship therapy with an accredited therapist

Second-line therapies

Oral therapies: 'daily or regular dosing on set days'

- Sildenafil
- Tadalafil
- Vardenafil

'Approved' intracavernosal injections

- Alprostadil (PGE1)

Transurethral pellets

- Alprostadil (MUSE®)

Third-line therapies

Unlicensed intracavernosal injections

- Trimix (papverine 30 mg/ml, phentolamine 1 mg/ml, alprostadil 10 µg/ml)
- Bimix (papverine 30 mg/ml, phentolamine 1 mg/ml – excessive response or penile pain with Trimix)

Fourth-line therapies

Penile implant surgery

Vascular reconstructive surgery

Education will help the patient, and help him to understand his ED and put it into context

50-year-old men with ED will be comforted by the thought that they are not alone and that around 50% of men of a similar age will experience ED at least some of the time.

Challenge and dispel any sexual myths that they might hold, for example, that they always ought to be able to get an erection on demand and 'give' their partner an orgasm. Through explanation, help the couple to understand each other's sexuality and sexual needs. Although it is a generalization, men tend to be more 'performance' orientated than women, judging sex to be a 'success' or 'failure' on the duration of the act and number of orgasms achieved. Women may also sometimes enjoy 'performance' in sex, but they are likely to value intimacy and closeness as important as the act itself.

Explanation: Explain the range of treatment options available, and those that you are able to offer within your practice.

Explain the whole range of treatment options and the patient's own treatment plan

Ensure that the patient fully understands your evaluation of his ED and which treatment options may be suitable for him, so that he can make an informed choice. Only the couple know which treatments will be compatible with their normal patterns of sexual behavior, so they should be allowed to make their own choice.

All practices should be able to offer basic sex education and behavioral advice, oral therapies, and vacuum tumescence devices (VTD). Do not assume that the couple are adequately informed about their sexual function; they may need very basic information about physiological and psychological processes, and the differences and similarities in response and interests in men and women. Behavioral advice is also very important; couples who have been affected by ED may have more or less completely ceased sharing physical intimacy [44]. Rediscovering physical intimacy and enjoying foreplay for its own sake may be an essential prelude to satisfactory intercourse [45].

Realistic expectations: Men should be encouraged to hold reasonable expectations for their sexual function and their ED therapy. Oral therapy should allow the vast majority to achieve hard erections, an important goal for most men with ED [46]. Erection hardness is the foundation stone upon which enjoyment of a better sexual experience is based. However, it is important to check out individual expectations and provide information about what can be realistically achieved. Be encouraging and enthusiastic, but temper this with realism; medication will not restore the full vigor, or body, of youth.

The aim of treatment is to enable a satisfactory sexual experience, not to restore the vigor of youth

Experience: Provide men with an adequate supply of medication to be used as frequently as they might reasonably desire; 8 – 12 doses of their chosen medication is a reasonable amount. Response to PDE5 inhibitors increases with successive doses, so men should be encouraged to persevere with medication for at least eight doses before abandoning it as ineffective [47]. Do not provide them with just four doses and tell them to come back in a month. Allow men the dignity to experiment in their own time, at the pace that they and their partner desire. After 5 years of ED, is it unreasonable to want to make love three times a week for a few weeks?

Once a regular pattern of erections and sexual behavior has been established, the frequency of intercourse is likely to settle down to the pre-ED value. There is no evidence that treating ED increases the frequency of sexual activity.

Ask men to make a follow-up appointment, preferably with their partner, once they have had the opportunity to use the treatment on a number of occasions. Around 8–12 attempts would be a reasonable number before evaluating their response.

Follow-up: All men provided with ED treatment should be offered follow-up consultations. It will be reassuring for them to know that they can come back and talk about their experience with ED therapy.

A significant proportion will not achieve a successful result first time. Some will give up before they have given the treatment a fair trial, while others will discover that there are other obstacles to their sexual expression than just ED. These issues should be addressed at follow-up. Some will move on to other therapies, or require referral, but many will need further education, explanation, and experience.

The importance of choice for individuals and couples

Consider the couple's choice of treatment, as it will probably reflect their sexual lifestyle

Individuals and couples will have their own preference for a particular therapy, as it may suit their own sexual lifestyle. The majority of men will select a PDE5 inhibitor as their first treatment of choice. Although the three currently available drugs in this class share a common mode of action, there are subtle pharmaco-kinetic differences among them that may be of importance to the couple that is unrecognized by the physician. The most obvious difference among them is that tadalafil has a much longer half-life and duration of effect than sildenafil and vardenafil (about 17 hours, compared with about 4 hours). Preference studies show conflicting results with each of the three drugs being most frequently preferred in different studies. However, it is clear that if men are given a choice of PDE5 inhibitor, they will express a preference for one. Perhaps the best approach is to allow men to try more than one and find which suits them best.

Couples will sometimes select other options as first choice: VTD and sex therapy are perfectly reasonable options, as their use is more-or-less without risk. Couples indicating a first preference for injections, transurethral pellets, or even implants should be carefully counseled about the risks and benefits of each option and encouraged to at least try lower-risk alternatives. Ultimately, the couple should be allowed to make an informed choice regarding their treatment option.

Providing a quality service

Continuing professional development: In order to be able to provide a high-quality service to men and couples affected by

ED, it is essential to maintain the appropriate knowledge and skills. This task should be approached in a holistic manner; to provide high-quality care, the physician needs to have a wide range of resources in sexology, urology, gynecology, and internal medicine.

While factual knowledge can be obtained from reading and personal study, skill acquisition is more difficult. Many doctors will find talking about sexual issues uncomfortable and struggle for appropriate language that is intelligible to clients without being too simplistic or too crude. Videos have been produced that illustrate the difficulties, but these are no substitute for practical experience. If you are unable to find a suitable skill acquisition course to attend, try working in pairs or threes with partners or local colleagues using case vignettes.

To begin with, discuss the case together, first exploring the clinical issues (which most people will feel more comfortable with) and then the communication issues. Draw up a list of words and expressions used to describe body parts and sexual behavior. What words might be used instead of penis, vagina, sexual drive and desire, erection, lubrication, masturbation, oral sex, intercourse, orgasm, and ejaculation?

Next, when you feel more comfortable, try role-playing the consultation. Take it in turns to act as patient and physician (and observer, if you work in threes). Focus on the communication issues to begin with. The person playing the patient should decide on what language to use and then use it consistently. The person playing the doctor should ensure that they understand the language used by repeating and seeking clarification. For example, if the patient says "I'm having trouble with my arousal", the doctor might ask "arousal?" or "can you explain to me what you mean by arousal?", or "by 'arousal', do you mean erection?"

Involving the extended healthcare team: Other members of your extended healthcare team may have the interest, knowledge and skills to contribute to the assessment and management of men

It is important to attain and maintain the appropriate knowledge and skills

Practice nurses may have valuable skills to offer in the assessment and treatment of ED with ED. In many countries, specialist nurses make a major contribution to ED and sexual healthcare; they are often seen by men as more approachable than doctors.

Practice administrative staff may feel uncomfortable about discussing sexual issues, and even find it uncomfortable to pass on information or make appointments for men with ED. Care should be taken to provide them with appropriate information, training, and support, so that they are able to deal with such matters in an open-minded and non-judgemental manner, respecting the confidentiality of affected individuals at all times.

FIRST-LINE INTERVENTIONS

- Basic sex education
- Oral therapies
- VTD
- Sexual and relationship therapy
- Treatment of ED after radical prostatectomy

Simple sex education

Basic sex education: This is the vital first step in effective treatment, leading to a successful outcome, in which the individual or couple can enjoy 'a satisfactory sexual experience', rather than just get erections. Do not underestimate its importance and do not omit it.

The importance of sex education should not be underestimated

Many men, including a large number of doctors, have a lamentably poor understanding of their sexuality and sexual function. Personal sex education is frequently delegated by parents to schools and tends to concentrate on reproductive biology, sexually transmitted diseases, and preventing unwanted pregnancy.

We are not educated in how to enjoy our own sexual feelings, or in understanding our partner's sexual needs and how we might best help them to fulfil them. Biology and Personal Development classes would probably be better attended if we did. Good role models are hard to find and, at present, most people learn from experience.

In addition to challenging the sexual myths mentioned earlier, helping men to understand the normal changes in sexual responsiveness that occur with aging is important. As men and women get older, changes occur in their attitudes toward, and experience of, sex. These changes should not always be seen as health problems, or 'getting old', but part of a natural development of their sexuality that began in childhood and will continue throughout their lives.

Men need to appreciate the normal changes in sexual responsiveness that occur with age

Older men often find that it takes longer for them to develop an erection. Young men often develop erections at the slightest sexually exciting thought or sight, which can be highly embarrassing for them. Older men, and their partners, often worry that they no longer get an erection when they think about sex or see their partner naked. They are convinced that this is a sign of serious illness or that they are becoming 'impotent'. This is incorrect.

Older men frequently require direct genital stimulation to achieve erection. It may take 5 or 10 minutes to develop, rather than seconds, as in their youth. In addition, they will often try and attempt intercourse before their erection is rigid, which is likely to result in penile buckling, loss of erection, and embarrassment. Drugs will probably deal with this problem, although achieving 'cure' through education must be the most desirable approach.

Couples should be encouraged to enjoy the changes that occur with age

Couples should be encouraged to enjoy the changes in sexual responsiveness that come with aging, rather than to simply fight against them. This does not mean that they must inevitably 'give up' on sharing sexual intimacy though.

If you feel that you are unable to address all of the necessary issues yourself, offer referral to a sexual and relationship therapist. However, some will refuse this and you may be their only source of appropriate sex education.

Oral therapies

Three PDE5 inhibitors are currently approved for use in North America and Europe: sildenafil (Viagra®, Pfizer), tadalafil (Cialis®, Lilly ICOS), and vardenafil (Levitra®, Bayer/GSK). Apomorphine (Uprima SL®, Abbott or Ixense®, Takeda), a dopaminergic agent, is available in Europe but not in the United States.

As couples' preferred sexual behaviors vary considerably, they should have the opportunity to choose their treatment, within the limitations imposed by concomitant medications or co-morbidity. These issues are discussed on Page 53.

A couple's sexual behavior may influence the choice of oral agent

Some couples habitually practice certain 'ritual' behaviors, with sex being more premeditated or planned. This may be as simple as normally having intercourse on a particular evening, or it may be quite complex, involving other sensory pleasures, such as food, alcohol, bathing, massage, and many other imaginative and enjoyable experiences practised to heighten desire and the intensity of the sexual experience.

PHOSPODIESTERASE TYPE-5 INHIBITORS

Mode of action: The PDE5 inhibitors (sildenafil, tadalafil and vardenafil) are highly selective inhibitors of the enzyme phosphodiesterase type-5. This enzyme is predominantly found in penile vascular smooth muscle and is responsible for the breakdown of cGMP. This is a chemical messenger and its production leads to smooth muscle relaxation and, in the case of penile vascular smooth muscle, erection (Figure 14).

Although some erections originate as a consequence of reflex pathways in the spinal cord, erection in response to sexual drive and desire begins in the mid-brain. It may occur in response to sexual thoughts (cognition), sights, sounds, smells, or touch.

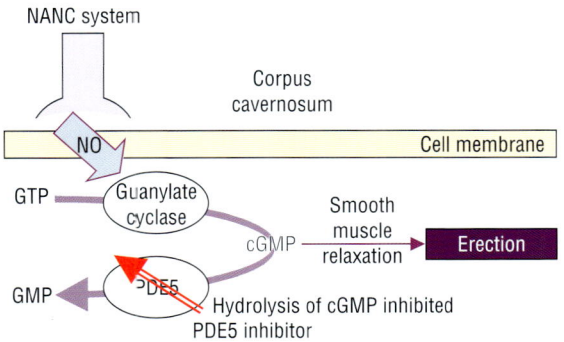

Figure 14. Mode of action for PDE5 inhibitors

Changes in dopaminergic activity in the mid-brain result in a change in the balance of genital autonomic tone, with a relative increase in parasympathetic activity promoting erection. Signals from the erectogenic centers of the mid-brain pass down the spinal cord to parasympathetic nuclei in the sacral cord. Efferent signals leave through the S2–S4 roots, and on through the nervi erigentes to the pelvic plexi and then the cavernous nerves, before finally reaching the penile vascular smooth muscle of the corpora cavernosa.

There is also a concurrent reduction in sympathetic activity, although this might not occur in men with performance anxiety-related ED. At the cellular level, parasympathetic nerve terminals adjacent to the penile vascular smooth muscle release a variety of neurotransmitters.

Nitric oxide generated by neuronal nitric oxide synthase (nNOS), is the erectogenic neurotransmitter that initiates erectile smooth muscle relaxation in the corpora cavernosa. It readily crosses the cell membrane into the smooth muscle fibers, where it activates guanylate cyclase, which converts guanosine triphosphate (GTP) to cGMP. The latter, in turn, causes smooth muscle relaxation, increased capacity of the penile vascular space, increased arterial inflow, tumescence, cavernosal veno-occlusion, and, finally, erection. Endothelium-derived nitric oxide synthase (eNOS) within the cavernosal endothelium generates further nitric oxide in response to shear stress within the erectile tissue, thus helping to maintain erection. Erection is terminated at orgasm by a shift in signaling, with a reduction in nitrergic nerve activity and increased sympathetic nerve activity, resulting in cavernosal and vascular smooth muscle contraction, disruption of the veno-occlusive mechanism, and detumescence.

This is a simplistic description of a very complex process, as there are other pathways and neurotransmitters involved, with considerable 'cross-talk' between them, further modifying erectile response. Other aspects of sexual response have different mechanisms. However, it is important to understand that PDE5 inhibitors prevent the degradation of cGMP and, thereby, enhance erectile responsiveness. It is essential to recall that these agents will not spontaneously provoke an erection and some sort of sexual stimulation is necessary for this to occur. If a man takes a PDE5 inhibitor and has no sexual stimulation during the next few hours, he will probably not get an erection at all.

> PDE5 inhibitors will only enhance erection if sexual stimulation has occurred

Use in practice: Because of differences in their pharmacokinetic properties, the three PDE5 inhibitors do offer couples different options.

Sildenafil: For most patients, the recommended dose is 50 mg taken, as needed, approximately 1 hour before sexual activity. However, sildenafil may be taken anywhere from 4 hours to 0.5 hour before sexual activity. Based on effectiveness and toleration, the dose may be increased to a maximum recommended dose of 100 mg or decreased to 25 mg. The maximum recommended dosing frequency is once per day [48].

Tadalafil: The recommended starting dose of tadalafil in most patients is 10 mg, taken prior to anticipated sexual activity. The dose may be increased to 20 mg or decreased to 5 mg, based on individual efficacy and tolerability. The maximum recommended dosing frequency is once per day in most patients. Tadalafil was shown to improve erectile function compared with placebo up to 36 hours following dosing. Therefore, when advising patients on optimal use this should be taken into consideration. It may be taken without regard to food [49].

Vardenafil: For most patients, the recommended starting dose of vardenafil is 10 mg, taken orally approximately 60 minutes before sexual activity. The dose may be increased to a maximum recommended dose of 20 mg or decreased to 5 mg based on efficacy and side effects The maximum recommended dosing frequency is once per day. Vardenafil can be taken with or without food [50].

With all the PDE5 inhibitors, the dose can be increased if it is not effective at the starting dose and reduced if adverse effects occur. There is a small increase in the prevalence of side effects at higher doses.

With these agents, the erection will be maintained whilst sexual stimulation continues and will usually go down after orgasm, or if stimulation ceases. If further stimulation occurs during the 'effective' period of the drug, the man may be able to get another erection. However, there is a 'refractory period' following orgasm, during which a man is unable to attain an erection despite sexual stimulation. In young men, this can be very short or even absent. In older men it can last for several hours.

It is common for men to take the drug too late, perhaps only remembering it when they go to bed. This will probably not allow adequate time for it to cause adequate PDE5 inhibition and it is likely to be ineffective. Explain to the couple that these agents must be given time to work but once taken will remain effective for at least 4–5 hours, or longer in the case of tadalafil.

Men should be encouraged to have at least 4 attempts before increasing dosage

There is a tendency for some men to give up after just one or two unsuccessful attempts. It is worth persevering with each dose and trying at least four times, on separate days, before changing to the next dose. No one should be considered a non-responder until they have tried such agents on at least eight occasions at the maximum tolerated dose.

Men should try at the maximum tolerated dose on 8 occasions before being considered non-responders

Once a given dose works reliably, it may be possible to reduce that dose and still achieve a useful effect.

Use in cardiovascular disease: All ED therapies, including PDE5 inhibitors, are contraindicated in severe unstable angina, recent myocardial infarction (within 4 weeks), recent stroke (within 6 months), severe heart failure, hypotension or uncontrolled hypertension, and other conditions where sexual activity is inadvisable.

There are published authoritative guidelines on the use of ED therapy in men with cardiovascular disease [18].

Drug interactions: There is a potentially dangerous interaction between all the PDE5 inhibitors and nitric oxide-donor drugs (which include nitrates and nicorandil) that can lead to severe hypotension; men should not take PDE5 inhibitors cocurrently with these drugs.

The concomitant use of PDE5 inhibitors and NO-donor drugs is *contraindicated*

Concomitant use of these agents with antihypertensive drugs (ACE inhibitors, beta-blockers, thiazide diuretics, and ATII-receptor blockers) is safe, although patients should be warned of possible decreases in blood pressure.

The PDE5 inhibitors share a common cytochrome system catabolic pathway (CYP3A4) with several other drugs (erythromycin, clarithromycin, itraconazole, ketaconazole, ritonavir, saquinavir, and indinavir) and concomitant use may increase plasma concentrations. Grapefruit juice is also an inhibitor of CYP3A4. Concomitant use with specific PDE5 inhibitors may be contraindicated, or require a reduction in dosage or frequency of administration; physicians should refer to the most recent manufacturer's Summary of Product Characteristics for further information.

Caution is necessary when PDE5 inhibitors are administered with alpha-blockers. Both PDE5 inhibitors and alpha-blockers are vasodilators. When used in combination, an additive effect on blood pressure may occur, lowering blood pressure significantly and leading to symptomatic hypotension. Consideration should be given to the following:

• Patients should be stable on alpha-blocker therapy prior to initiating a PDE5 inhibitor. Patients who demonstrate hemodynamic instability on alpha-blocker therapy alone are at increased risk of symptomatic hypotension with concomitant use of PDE5 inhibitors.

- In those patients who are stable on alpha-blocker therapy, PDE5 inhibitors should be initiated at the lowest recommended starting dose.

- In those patients already taking an optimized dose of PDE5 inhibitor, alpha-blocker therapy should be initiated at the lowest dose. A stepwise increase in alpha-blocker dose may be associated with further lowering of blood pressure in patients taking a PDE5 inhibitor.

Other information: Special care needs to be taken when prescribing PDE5 inhibitors for men with conditions that might predispose them to have a prolonged erection, such as leukemia, multiple myeloma, and sickle cell disease.

Caution is advised in the use of PDE5 inhibitors in men with Peyronie's disease, probably because men with this condition were excluded from the pivotal studies used in licensing applications. It is difficult to conceive how these men with Peyronie's disease would be at any additional risk from the use of PDE5 inhibitors, other than that those with deformity causing severe impairment of the veno-occlusive mechanism may not respond as well.

The administration of PDE5 inhibitors should be avoided in cases of severe hepatic or renal impairment, or only prescribed on specialist advice.

Adverse effects: PDE5 inhibitors are well tolerated by most men. The common reported adverse effects include headache, facial flushing, mild dyspepsia, and nasal congestion. A comparison of the adverse events for the three PDE5 inhibitors is shown in the table overleaf.

Transient changes in color vision have been reported with sildenafil and, less frequently, with vardenafil. The use of all these agents is contraindicated in men with hereditary degenerative retinal disorders. Transient myalgia and back pain have been reported with tadalafil.

PDE5 INHIBITORS			
	Sildenafil	Tadalafil	Vardenafil
Dosing	25/50/100 mg	10/20 mg	5/10/20 mg
Time to onset	~1 hour	~1 hour	~1 hour
Duration of effect	4–6 hours	24 hours	4–6 hours
Side effects			
Headache	16%	14%	16%
Dizziness	-	2%	3%
Flushing	10%	4%	12%
Nasal congestion	4%	4%	3%
Dyspepsia (mild)	7%	12%	4%
Back pain	-	7%	-
Myalgia	-	6%	-
Changes in color vision	3%	-	-

Contraindications

- Nitric oxide-donor drugs (e.g. nitrates, nicorandil)
- In situations where sexual activity is inadvisable: severe unstable angina, recent MI or stroke, or severe heart failure /hypotension/ uncontrolled hypertension
- Known hypersensitivity to an ingredient of the formulation
- Hereditary degenerative retinal disorders

Cautious use

- Conditions predisposing to priapism (leukemia, multiple myeloma, sickle cell disease)
- Peyronie's disease
- Severe renal / hepatic impairment

Potential drug interactions

- Clarithromycin, saquinavir, ketaconazole, grapefruit juice
- Ritonavir, itraconazole, indinavir
- Erythromycin
- Alpha-blockers

APOMORPHINE

Mode of action: Apomorphine is a centrally acting drug for the treatment of ED; it is not approved in the United States, although it is available in Europe. CNS control of sexual function is thought to be maintained through a balance of inhibitory and excitatory systems, influenced by androgens and by erectogenic stimuli from centers of the brain concerned with sight, sound, smell, touch, and cognition. A variety of neurotransmitters are involved but, simplistically, the primary neurotransmitter of central sexual inhibition is serotonin, and of central sexual excitation, dopamine. Apomorphine activates dopamine D2 receptors in the hypothalamus and has the potential to both initiate an erection and enhance responsiveness to erectogenic stimuli (Figure 15).

Apomorphine should be taken sublingually. It will probably be ineffective if swallowed

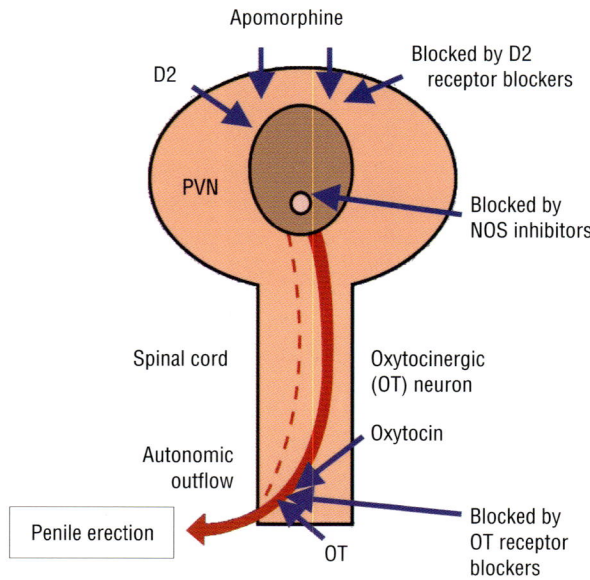

Figure 15. Mode of action for apomorphine

Use in practice: Proper counseling about the use of any therapy is vital to a successful outcome, but particularly so with ED therapy. Apomorphine is taken sublingually and it is essential that the patient be told to pop it under the tongue, and to allow it to dissolve slowly rather than suck or swallow it. If it is swallowed, it will probably be ineffective, because of the very high proportion of drug metabolized on the first pass through the liver. The 2-mg tablet is pentagonal, and the 3-mg, triangular.

The response rate to apomorphine is significantly less than for the PDE5 inhibitors. A randomized, placebo-controlled, crossover study comparing apomorphine 3 mg with sildenafil 50 mg in the treatment of ED of mixed etiology and severity reported attempts resulting in erections firm enough for intercourse in 44% of men taking apomorphine and 85% of men taking sildenafil [51]. One of the proposed advantages of apomorphine is its relatively rapid onset of action. Clinical trial evidence shows that 71% of responders will achieve an erection within 20 minutes of putting the tablet in their mouths. Apomorphine can be taken once every 8 hours.

All men should start with one dose of the 2-mg presentation. They should increase this to 3 mg if the starting dose is well tolerated. Only 15% of men will respond to 2 mg, but dose titration will reduce the risk of users suddenly experiencing unwanted side effects. It is important not to label men 'non-responders' because they do not respond to the first few doses of apomorphine. Some men will give up after just one or two unsuccessful attempts with oral therapy. It should be explained that there is often considerable general and performance anxiety surrounding the use of a new ED medication, which will tend to inhibit erectile responsiveness.

In addition, if men are paying for apomorphine themselves, they may not understand why it is necessary to keep taking a drug that doesn't work first time. They should be advised to

> With apomorphine 71% of responders will achieve an erection within 20 minutes

> A trial of at least 8 attempts with apomorphine is suggested

take at least eight doses of 3 mg, in an appropriate environment and with adequate sexual stimulation, before deciding whether or not it is effective for them (Figure 16).

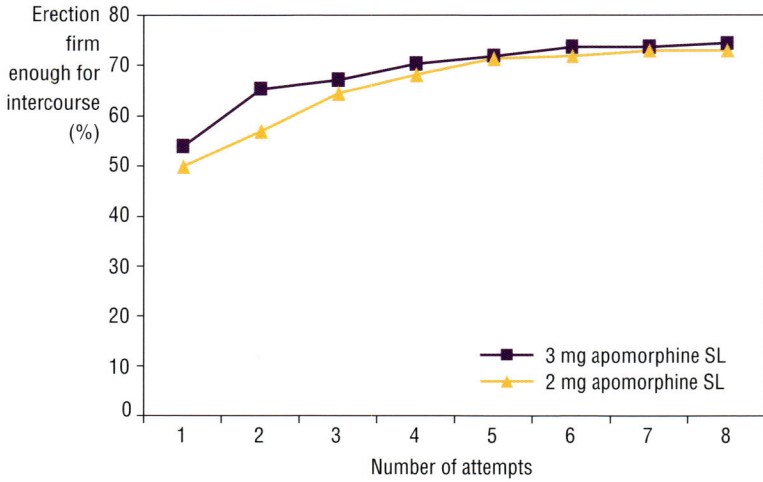

Figure 16. Effect of sequential doses on treatment response with apomorphine

As with PDE5 inhibitors, non-responders should be closely questioned about how they took the drug, how many doses they had taken, and under what circumstances. Genuine non-responders should be offered appropriate alternative therapies.

Adverse effects: Because of its relative selectivity for the dopamine D2 receptor, apomorphine is reasonably well-tolerated and there is a low incidence of dopaminergic side effects, such as nausea, vomiting (probably D3 receptors), and hypotension (probably D5 receptors).

In trials of 2-mg and 3-mg tablets, 6.8% of men reported nausea, 6.7% reported headaches, 4.4% reported dizziness and 0.2% reported syncope. The reported nausea was usually mild and tended to disappear with repeated use. More than 90% of those men who reported syncope experienced premonitory vasovagal symptoms. Men should be warned not to drive for 2 hours after taking apomorphine, although this is unlikely to be a significant disadvantage for the majority of users. It is sensible to advise users to avoid all potentially dangerous activities, such as climbing ladders or operating machinery, for the same period.

Use in cardiovascular disease: All ED therapies, including apomorphine, are contraindicated in men with severe unstable angina, recent MI (within 4 weeks), severe heart failure or hypotension, and other conditions where sexual activity is inadvisable.

It should be used with caution in men with a history of uncontrolled hypertension, known hypotension, postural hypotension, or those with compromised renal or hepatic function. Apomorphine can be used with caution in men taking anti-hypertensives or nitric oxide donor medications, such as nitrates and nicorandil.

There are published authoritative guidelines on the use of ED therapy in men with cardiovascular disease [18].

Drug interactions: Special care must be taken in prescribing apomorphine to men taking other drugs that act on dopamine receptors, such as antipsychotics and antiemetics, Apomorphine is a dopamine D2 receptor agonist and most antipsychotics are dopamine D2 receptor antagonists. It seems sensible that if a combination is prescribed, then the patient should be followed up more carefully for the first weeks of treatment. There is no evidence that the sublingual presentation of apomorphine has any effect on antipsychotic therapy but there may be theoretical risk of precipitating a relapse of psychotic illness. It should not be used in combination with sildenafil or other ED therapies.

Men should be warned not to drive for 2 hours after taking apomorphine

69

APOMORPHINE			
Side effects			
• Nausea (6.8%) • Headache (6.7%)		• Dizziness (4.4%) • Syncope (0.2%)	
Contraindications			
• Known hypersensitivity to an ingredient of the formulation			
• In situations where sexual activity is inadvisable: severe unstable angina, recent MI (within 4 weeks), and severe heart failure / hypotension			
Cautious use			
• Uncontrolled hypertension			
• Postural hypotension			
• Compromised renal / hepatic function			
• Patients taking anti-hypertensive medications			
• Men taking nitric oxide-donor medications (e.g. nitrates, nicorandil)			
Possible drug interactions			
• Antipsychotics			
• Antiemetics			
• PDE5 inhibitors			

Vacuum tumescence devices

Mode of action: VTD were developed in the 1960s and were the first truly effective treatment for ED. To produce an erection, the flaccid penis is placed in a cylinder, with one end connected to a vacuum pump and the other pressed firmly against the abdominal wall, usually with an aqueous lubricant jelly, to obtain a pressure seal. The pump is operated and the pressure in the cylinder is reduced to below atmospheric pressure. Blood is drawn into the corpora cavernosa of the penis by retrograde flow through the venous system, leading to tumescence and, eventually, erection. Once the penis is erect, a constriction ring, previously loaded around the base of the cylinder, is slipped over the penile shaft, close to the abdominal wall. The ring should be just tight enough to trap blood within the corpora cavernosa, thus maintaining erection (Figure 17).

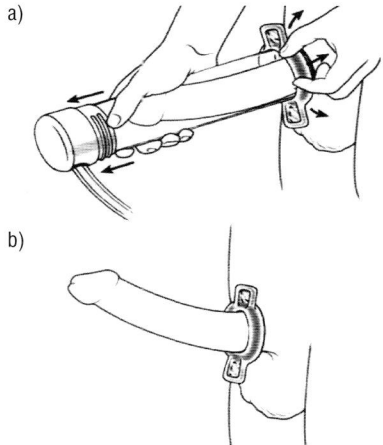

a)

b)

Figure 17.
Use of vacuum
erection device

The pressure within the cylinder is then allowed to return to atmospheric and then removed. The penis should remain erect for as long as the ring is left in place. The ring must be removed within 30 minutes of application.

Use in practice: VTD are highly effective in producing erections, even where other pharmacological treatments have failed. Some people are attracted by a method that does not involve the use of drugs.

If the couple select a VTD as their treatment of first choice, most will be very satisfied with it; a continuation rate of 81% at 6 months has been reported [52]. Those who use VTD as a last resort are far more likely to be dissatisfied with it [53]. Modern devices and ring systems are simpler and more comfortable to use, and may result in greater acceptability. However, this is very dependent on how the device is presented to them by the

VTD can be effective in producing erections even when pharmacological therapies have failed

71

physician. If it is presented in a positive manner, acceptance and user satisfaction is far more likely. It is important not to convey any of one's own negative attitudes toward the VTD, which one might personally perceive as cumbersome and unattractive.

If you are planning to offer men VTD, it is important to have one available for demonstration. Some manufacturers may be willing to provide one free of charge or at a discounted price to health professionals. They also produce a range of support materials, including instructional videos. VTD cannot be adequately sterilized, so it is inadvisable to loan patients devices for home trials. It is advisable to ask them to purchase the device and bring it back to the office, so that they can be shown how it works. Take time to show them how to obtain a good pressure seal and how to operate the pump. Users should not be too vigorous in pumping, as they might cause bruising or rupture of small subcutaneous veins. Having been shown how to use the device successfully in the office, they will be far more confident when trying it at home. VTD work for just about everyone; patients who claim the device does not work should have their technique of application carefully reviewed in the office. It is more likely that use of the device is unacceptable to the man or his partner.

The constriction ring worn with the VTD commonly restricts ejaculation

Other information: Men using VTD commonly report restriction of ejaculation, due to the necessity of wearing a constriction ring. Whilst this is harmless, it may be uncomfortable or unacceptable for other reasons. Clearly, the constriction ring needs to be tight enough to trap blood in the corpora and this can also lead to discomfort or loss of sensation, perhaps due to transient neuropraxia. Because of the venous stasis, the surface temperature of the penis may drop a few degrees and women sometimes complain that their partner's penis feels cold. As mentioned above, over-vigorous pumping may lead to bruising, as can application of the constriction ring, particularly in anticoagulated men.

As the penis is only erect in the segment distal to the constriction ring, with the base and penile crura remaining flaccid, it will 'hinge' around the ring. In practice, the penis may need to be lifted manually to facilitate penetration, as it will tend to point downward at all times.

Finally, it is essential that the ring is removed within 30 minutes of application; otherwise there is a risk of causing ischemic damage to the penis. In extreme cases, say if the man fell asleep with the ring in place for several hours, this might eventually lead to penile necrosis. Such reports are, happily, rare.

The constriction ring should be removed within 30 minutes to avoid the risk of ischemic damage

Sexual and relationship therapy

Sexual and relationship therapy is an important clinical discipline, which requires specific training. It is far more than an extension of general counseling. Practices that do not have such a therapist available 'in-house' will have to refer appropriate individuals or couple to an accredited sexual and relationship therapist.

Sexual and relationship therapy may be considered a specialized branch of psychotherapy. It usually involves the use of cognitive-behavioral techniques aimed at the relief of the individual's (or couple's) sexual dysfunction, involving sex education and the practice of sexual and communication tasks as a part of the treatment process, with regular feedback sessions with the therapist.

Sexual and relationships therapy is distinct from psychoanalytical or marital therapy

It differs from psychoanalytic treatment, which attempts to resolve unconscious conflicts that might be causing dysfunction, and marital therapy, which attempts to improve a couple's general relationship quality by helping them to resolve unrecognized conflicts. Psychoanalytic and marital therapy techniques may be used by a therapist, but are not at the core of sexual and relationship therapy.

Sexual and relationship therapy is generally considered effective treatment for ED, although this has not been unequivocally demonstrated in trials. A 'success rate' of around 60% is commonly quoted, although the size and durability of effect is uncertain. It is likely that older men with complete ED, diabetes and severe vascular disease are less likely to respond than younger men with intermittent or situational ED, and no concomitant medical problems.

Younger men with intermittent or situational ED are more likely to respond

Sexual and relationship therapy is effective in the treatment of premature ejaculation, delayed or anorgasmia (for which there is good research evidence), and vaginismus.

It may also be beneficial in desire disorders, although those affected should also have an appropriate endocrine and medical assessment.

Managing 'non-responders'

Not everyone will respond to, or find acceptable in practice, their first choice of therapy. However, it is important to check that the chosen therapy has been used according to your recommendations before labeling someone a non-responder. It is often quite revealing to ask the following questions:

- How was the treatment used or taken, and what happened?
- How many times has it been tried?
- How many of those tries were followed by an attempt at intercourse?
- What was the partner's view of the treatment?
- How does the user feel about the treatment?

Genuine non-responders should be re-assessed. In particular, it is important to check your working diagnosis of ED, rather than a relationship problem or premature ejaculation. It is not that uncommon for men to complain of 'impotence' when, in fact, their partner refuses to have intercourse with them.

Managing non-responders to oral therapy: A significant proportion of men report failure to respond to oral therapies when they are first prescribed. Sometimes this is due to failure to follow physician instructions on drug use (or physician failure to explain the treatment adequately), and around one-third of apparent PDE5 inhibitor non-responders may become responders if adequately re-instructed in correct drug use [54,55]. Dose escalation and stressing the need for adequate stimulation may also salvage some non-responders. Recent research suggests that non-responders using 'on-demand' dosing can be salvaged by daily or regular dosing with PDE5 inhibitors [56,57]. Continued non-responders should have testosterone levels evaluated, as normalizing testosterone may salvage some non-responders.

Treatment of ED after radical prostatectomy

The majority of men who have had a radical prostatectomy will have ED for at least a limited period, and some will have permanent problems that are resistant to oral therapies. They present a particularly challenging group to treat, and management strategies are still evolving.

The likelihood of a man experiencing post-radical prostatectomy ED is influenced by his pre-operative potency, his age (ED is more likely if over 65), and the achievement of intra-operative nerve preservation (ED is more likely if one or both cavernous nerves are sacrificed).

Pre-operative counseling about sexual and erectile function should be included in the routine care of men facing radical prostatectomy, and it is preferable to involve their partners too. The type of post-operative treatment regiments offered should be discussed. If possible, they should have pre-operative treatment for any pre-existing ED; this will not only allow them to enjoy sexual intimacy but also give the physician an idea of 'baseline' erectile function.

Traditionally, men with ED after radical prostatectomy would be offered the same treatment regiment as men with ED resulting from other causes (i.e. on-demand use of PDE5 inhibitors introduced at a time of the patient's choosing after surgery). Pioneering research by Montorsi and colleagues in the late 1990s suggested that men who were restored to potency by the early post-operative introduction of intracavernosal injection therapy had a better chance of recovering normal erectile function, without medication [58]. This suggested that an 'erection rehabilitation program' after radical prostatectomy might offer men a better chance of recovering normal erectile function.

Further work by Mulhall and colleagues has shown that the early introduction of oral therapy may confer a similar benefit in men able to achieve at least a partial erection response to sildenafil 100 mg [59]. Responsive patients were instructed to use sildenafil to obtain an erection three times a week. Non-responders were offered intracavernous injections as an alternative but were re-challenged with sildenafil every 4 months after surgery. Subsequent responders were offered transfer to the oral therapy regime. There was a statistically significant difference ($p < 0.001$) in the percentage of patients who could obtain a functional erection without medication at 18 months after surgery between those who had participated in the rehabilitation program (52%) and those who had not (19%). Although there are methodological flaws in this study, which were acknowledged by the authors, this striking difference has resulted in many centers offering similar rehabilitation programs to their patients.

It has been speculated that the mechanism by which this apparent benefit is achieved is through maintaining intermittent cavernous re-perfusion and oxygenation, resulting in a reduction in smooth muscle apoptosis. This prevents disruption of the veno-occlusive mechanism of erection until cavernous nerve function has recovered adequately for normal erections to resume. Further research is necessary to confirm these interesting findings and to identify the optimal rehabilitation treatment regiment. Three erections a week was an arbitrary choice of convenience; normally potent men will have far more frequent nocturnal and stimulated erections. There is also the issue of cost, inconvenience to the patient, and the possibility of treatment-related adverse effects with oral therapy or, more likely, injection therapy. In any event, it seems that rehabilitation programs may offer the hope of better recovery of erections in this difficult-to-treat group of patients.

SECOND-LINE AND FURTHER INTERVENTIONS

Second-line interventions

- Approved intracavernosal injection therapy
- Transurethral therapy

Most physicians with an interest in sexual medicine and ED will offer transurethral or intracavernosal therapy. The techniques for preparing and administering such treatments are fairly straightforward but it is much more challenging to actually teach another person how to do it. If you are interested in offering these treatments, it would be sensible to spend some time with a health professional experienced in teaching patients these techniques, as you will have to develop teaching as well as clinical skills.

Intracavernosal injection therapy

Alprostadil (prostaglandin E_1 [PGE_1]) is the most widely-used injectable agent in Europe and is the only approved agent in the United States.

Mode of action: With injection therapy, the drug is delivered directly into the corpora cavernosa (Figure 18). Only a single injection is necessary, as numerous venous channels intimately link the paired corpora and the drug is rapidly distributed throughout.

Once in the corpora cavernosa, alprostadil binds to specific receptors on the smooth muscle cell membrane, which, in turn, will activate intracellular adenylate cyclase. This enzyme converts adenosine triphosphate (ATP) to cyclic adenosine monophosphate, which, in turn, causes a rise in the intracellular calcium concentration and smooth muscle relaxation. This

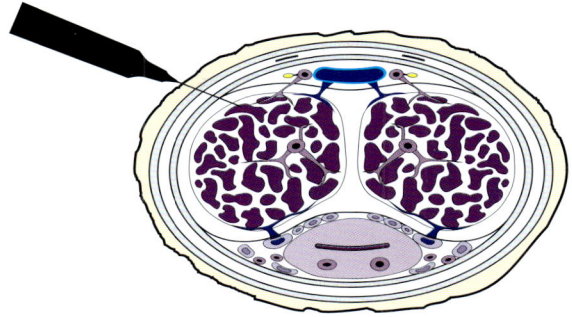

Figure 18.
Intracavernosal
injection therapy

leads to an increase in the capacity of the penile vascular space, increased arterial inflow, tumescence, and, finally, erection.

Use in practice: Alprostadil is usually presented as alprostadil powder and a dilutant, which are mixed just before injection. Mixing is necessary as alprostadil is not stable in solution for the prolonged periods required for storage and distribution in the pharmaceutical industry.

The first injections of alprostadil should be administered in the physician's office by medically trained personnel. Injections are given into the dorso-lateral aspect of the penile shaft, proximal to the coronal sulcus and glans, avoiding the midline and any obvious superficial veins. Erection will develop 5–20 minutes after injection and is intended to last for around 1 hour. Erection duration is dose related and administering too high a dose may result in priapism. Men should start at a low dose and titrate this according to response and erection duration. The US product label recommends a starting dose of 2.5 μg for most men and 1.25 μg for men with pure neurogenic ED (spinal cord injury) should start on 2.5 μg. The method for dose escalation is discussed in detail in the product label, which should be studied carefully by prescribing physicians [60]. Some individuals are very sensitive to small dose increases. The response rate for alprostadil administered as a single agent is in excess of 75%.

Erection will occur within 5–20 minutes and should last for about 1 hour

The response rate for intracavernosal alprostadil is over 75%

79

The key to successful treatment is the provision of good training, support, and follow-up to users. Only practices that are prepared to offer this should offer injection therapy. Injections should not be administered more frequently than once in 24 hours or more than three times each week.

Other information: Penile pain during or immediately after injection has been reported by 10–31% of users. This effect is not only due to the act of injection, but at least in part to the drug or its dilutant as well. Bruising can occur but can also be largely prevented by good injection technique. If the injection is inadvertently given on the ventral surface of the penis, it is possible to inject the drug into the urethral lumen, resulting in it escaping through the urethral meatus, sometimes accompanied by a little bleeding. Although usually harmless, this can be disconcerting to users. Rarely, users may become hypotensive, feeling dizzy, or light-headed after injection. This may be due to a systemic effect of the drug or to a vasovagal reaction to the injection itself.

Men should be warned that this treatment might cause penile fibrosis

Penile fibrosis (Peyronie's disease) is more common in men using intracavernosal injection, whatever drug is used. Men should be warned that they might develop this condition as a consequence of injection therapy, not least for medico-legal reasons. The risk of developing the problem may be reduced by using good injection technique and by varying the injection site. More frequent users are at greater risk. Those affected should be advised to stop using the drug and to seek medical advice at the next available opportunity.

Priapism is a dose-related adverse event and should only occur in 1:250 users if a careful dose titration policy is followed

Priapism, a persistent, prolonged and painful erection in the absence of sexual stimulation, can develop following intracavernosal injection of alprostadil. This is a dose-related effect and initiating therapy at a low dose and gradually titrating it according to response and erection duration will reduce the risk. If such a policy is adopted, the incidence is low, affecting less than 1 in 250 users. Men who experience an erection lasting more than 4 hours following injection should be considered to have priapism. It is a urological emergency and all men using intracavernosal injection therapy should be given written guidance on what to do if this occurs. In most circumstances, this will involve attendance at the prescribing physician's office or the local emergency room.

Transurethral therapy

MUSE® (alprostadil) is the only licensed preparation for transurethral therapy.

Mode of action: The mode of action of alprostadil is described earlier, in the section on intracavernosal injection therapy. Alprostadil is delivered into the penile urethra and is absorbed through the epithelium into the venous channels of the corpus spongiosum. It reaches the vascular smooth muscle of the corpora cavernosa by retrograde flow through emissary veins, encouraged by penile massage at the time of administration. Much of the dose is lost into the pelvic veins, however.

The patient should sit or stand during administration, to minimize absorption of alprostadil into the systemic circulation

Use in practice: In the form of MUSE, alprostadil is delivered as a small pellet, mounted on a fine plastic introducer. It is important that the man is either sitting or standing during administration, as laying flat results in more of the drug escaping to the general venous circulation. In some men, the addition of a penile constriction ring may improve response.

It should be inserted into the urethra immediately after micturition, the moisture facilitating insertion and the dissolution of the pellet (Figure 19). The penis should then be vigorously massaged between the palms of both hands for a few minutes.

In responders, an erection will develop in 15–20 minutes, and will last for up to 1 hour. The response rate in home use is around 45%. MUSE should not be administered more frequently than twice in 24 hours, or more than seven times each week.

The most frequent side effects are penile pain (30%) and minor urethral bleeding

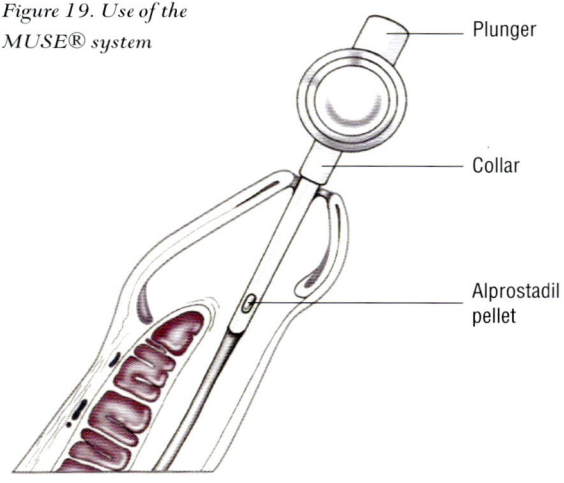

Figure 19. Use of the MUSE® system

Plunger

Collar

Alprostadil pellet

Other information: About one-third of men using MUSE report penile pain at the time of administration, with about 10% experiencing continuing pain after administration. While this is harmless, it can be distressing and is a common reason for discontinuation. Some men report aching, flushing, or dilatation of leg veins following administration. Occasionally, men report urethral bleeding following administration, probably due to minor urethral trauma. There have been rare reports of penile fibrosis (Peyronie's disease) and priapism. Men who experience an erection lasting more than 4 hours after administration of MUSE should be considered to have priapism. Although rare with MUSE, it is a urological emergency and all men should be given written guidance on what to do if this occurs. In most circumstances, this will involve attendance at the prescribing physician's office or the local emergency room.

Interestingly, there have also been reports from partners of vaginal irritation or discomfort. MUSE should not be used with a pregnant partner.

THIRD-LINE INTERVENTIONS

Third-line therapies mostly involve the use of unapproved drugs or unapproved combinations of approved and unapproved drugs. They are the province of the sexual medicine specialist, who must take great care to discuss with patients their potential risks and benefits, their regulatory status, and medico-legal implications of their use.

Combination drug therapies

There has been long experience with combinations of different drugs used for intracavernosal injection, although they are unapproved and there is limited evidence for their efficacy and safety. 'Trimix' (papverine 30 mg/ml, phentolamine 1 mg/ml, alprostadil 10 μg/ml) and 'bimix' (papverine 30 mg/ml, phentolamine 1 mg/ml) are widely used at varying doses in urological practice in the United States, although less so in Europe. Bimix is offered where the alprostadil component of Trimix causes bothersome penile pain. These combinations have been reported as effective when alprostadil has failed as a single agent. Papaverine was first reported as an effective pharmacotherapy for ED in 1982 [61]; with the addition of phentolamine, Bimix has been used since 1983, with Trimix being used rather more recently.

FOURTH-LINE INTERVENTIONS
(only provided in secondary care)

- Penile implant surgery
- Vascular reconstructive surgery

Only a small proportion of men fail to respond to modern medical therapy. Almost all of them could achieve erection through surgery, although, in practice, few choose to do so.

83

Surgical treatment should be considered in men who have failed to respond to existing medical therapies, or who find them unacceptable. Patients who select a prosthesis as their preferred treatment option are usually highly motivated.

Penile implant surgery

Mode of action: The basic principle of implant surgery is to replace the ineffective corpora cavernosa with a semi-rigid prosthesis that provides adequate penile rigidity for enjoyable sexual activity, usually vaginal penetration [62]. By necessity, the internal structure of the corpora is destroyed to make space for the implant, rendering future attempts at medical therapy more-or-less impossible. The size of prosthesis can be adjusted to fit the patient's intracorporal space. Some patients request a larger prosthesis in the hope that they can increase their penile length. Insertion of a longer prosthesis than that which the corpora can accommodate may be disastrous, failing to properly inflate. The surgeon takes great care to ensure that only the correct-sized prosthesis is used. As with all therapies for ED, careful counseling and assessment are essential for a satisfactory outcome.

Types of prosthesis: There are three classes of penile prosthesis: hydraulic (inflatable), semi-rigid, and mechanical. There are a range of inflatable prostheses from different manufacturers, in two- and three-part formats. The surgeon will select the appropriate device for the particular patient, as some are more suitable in specific circumstances (such as after cavernosal fibrosis) than others. Some devices are antibiotic coated, to reduce the risk of infection. Infection rates with modern surgical techniques are low (1–3%), although it can still be disastrous when it occurs, necessitating a salvage procedure or removal of the prosthesis.

The prosthetic cylinders are placed within the corpora and are inflated by the patient using a scrotal pump when penile rigidity is desired. The advantage of this rather complex and expensive device is that the appearance of the flaccid genitalia is quite normal and erections are more physiologic. This may be essential for younger and more active men, to enable them to lead a more normal sexual life. Prosthesis failure is now much less common than when the devices were introduced 30 years ago. Failure rates in the range of 5–10% within the first 5 years are to be expected and when counseling patients, these figures should be quoted.

Malleable, semi-rigid, and mechanical implants are inserted directly into the corpora (Figure 20). As their name suggests, the penis will remain in a permanent state of semi-rigidity. As the rods are malleable (rather like a smoker's pipe cleaner), the penis can be bent upward when needed for sexual activity and downward at other times. This type of implant is not always cosmetically acceptable to men who wear swimming trunks, sports clothing,

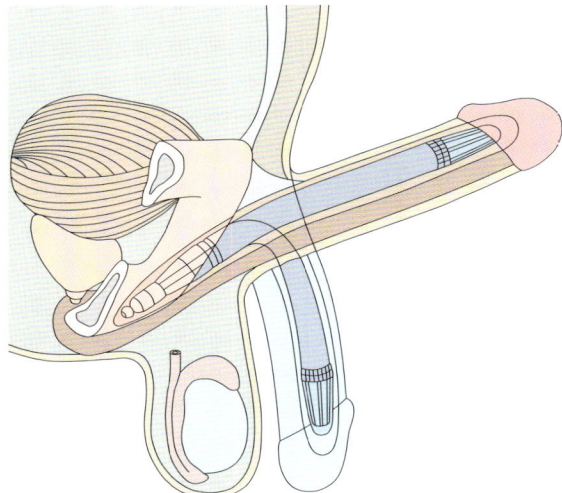

Figure 20. Semi-rigid rod prosthesis

or other relatively tight clothes, such as jeans. These relatively simple devices are much less prone to mechanical failure.

Patient satisfaction: Patients who have successful implantation of a penile prosthesis are reported to have a high rate of satisfaction with their treatment outcome, greater than 90% in several studies. Men who have implants after radical prostatectomy or Peyronie's disease report lower satisfaction rates, although these are still above 85% [63].

Vascular reconstructive surgery

Surgical techniques have been developed to improve arterial inflow to, and reduce venous outflow from, the penis in attempts to improve erection, but they are still investigational. Studies have shown that the results of such surgery, except in highly selected cases such as recently acquired, post-traumatic arterial obstruction, are deeply disappointing.

Arterial surgery: As erection is essentially a neurovascular event, it seems logical that some form of arterial revascularization procedure may be effective in restoring erectile function. This has proved to be the case in younger men with a single arterial lesion sustained as a result of pelvic or perineal trauma. However, revascularization is not effective in the long-term for men with atherosclerosis or diabetes.

Venous surgery: Erection is maintained because the high pressure within the corpora cavernosa compresses the emissary veins passing through the tunica albuginea, restricting venous drainage and preventing detumescence. It has been postulated that ligation of various veins in the penis might be an effective treatment for ED. However, the results have been deeply disappointing. Venous surgery has now been largely abandoned as a treatment for ED, other than for men who have sustained abnormal arterio-venous or veno-venous communications as a result of trauma.

SUMMARY

Sex is a central part of the human experience and to deny this is to deny our humanity. Whilst some people make a choice to remain celibate and clearly enjoy wholly fulfilling lives, for the vast majority, sex remains important to them throughout their adult lives.

Traditionally, ED has been the almost-exclusive preserve of the urologist and psychiatrist. In the past 20 years, a new discipline of sexual medicine has evolved, as our scientific understanding of human sexuality has evolved. Urologists still play an important leadership role in this field and many are amongst the increasing ranks of 'Sexual Physicians', offering holistic care to men and women with sexual concerns. They use biomedical and psychotherapeutic techniques and have skills in psychology, different disciplines of internal medicine, and gynecology, as well as urology.

Treating ED effectively and well is a tremendously satisfying professional experience. Almost every individual and couple will benefit from the support, education and therapeutic interventions offered. Even if they are unable to fulfil their expectations of treatment, the therapeutic experience will have informed them and will often have enabled them to better adapt to their situation.

Physicians who treat ED and other sexual problems are not just in the business of helping people have sex. They promote relationships; they help people to communicate more effectively and to share intimacy. They don't just treat men's penises, they help couples and families. There are demonstrable social benefits from treating ED and sexual problems; the few reports of adverse social outcomes are far outweighed by the positive social benefits to millions of people worldwide.

REFERENCES

1. Wagner G, Claes H, Costa P, *et al*. A shared care approach to the management of erectile dysfunction in the community. *Int J Impot Res* 2002;14:189–94.

2. Lue TF, Giuliano F, Montorsi F, *et al*. Summary of the recommendations on sexual dysfunctions in men. *J Sex Med* 2004;1:6–23.

3. Kinsella K, Gist YJ. *Gender and Aging. US Department of Commerce, Economics and Statistics Administration*. Bureaux of the Census, IB/98-2, Issued October 1998.

4. Fisher WA, Meryn S, Sand M, *et al*. Communication about erectile dysfunction among men with ED, partners of men with ED, and physicians; the Strike Up a Conversation study (part I). *JMHG* 2005;2:64–78.

5. Fisher WA, Meryn S, Sand M, *et al*. Communication about erectile dysfunction among men with ED, partners of men with ED, and physicians; the Strike Up a Conversation study (part II). *JMHG* 2005;2:309.e1–309.e12.

6. Jackson G, Rosen RC, Kloner RA, *et al*. The second Princeton consensus on sexual dysfunction and cardiac risk: new guidelines for sexual medicine. *J Sex Med* 2006;3:28–36.

7. Hirsch M, Donatucci C, Glina S, *et al*. Standards for clinical trials in male sexual dysfunction: erectile dysfunction and rapid ejaculation. *J Sex Med* 2004;1:87–91.

8. Feldman HA, Goldstein I, Hatzichristou DG, *et al*. Impotence and its medical and psychosocial correlates: results of the Massachusetts Male Aging Study. *J Urol* 1994;151:54–61.

9. Sommer F, Schulze W. Treating erectile dysfunction by endothelial rehabilitation with phosphodiesterase 5 inhibitors. *World J Urol* 2005;23:385–92.

10. Carson CC, Kirby RS, Goldstein I, *et al*. *Textbook of Erectile Dysfunction*. Oxford: ISIS Medical Media, 1999.

11. Andersson KE, Wagner G. Physiology of penile erection. *Physiol Rev* 1995;75:191–236.

12. Traish AM, Guay AT. Are androgens critical for penile erections in humans? Examining the clinical and preclinical evidence. *J Sex Med* 3:382–407.

13. Deveci S, Palese M, Parker M, *et al*. Erectile function profiles in men with Peyronie's disease. *J Urol* 2006;175:1807–11.

14. Mulhall JP, Schiff J, Guhring P. An analysis of the natural history of Peyronie's disease. *J Urol* 2006;175:2115–8.

15. Nehra A, Goldstein I, Pabby A, *et al*. Mechanisms of venous leakage: a prospective clinicopathological correlation of corporeal function and structure. *J Urol* 1996;156:1320–9.

16. Patrick DL, Althof SE, Pryor JL, *et al*. Premature ejaculation: an observational study of men and their partners. *J Sex Med* 2005;2:358–67.

17. Kesteren P, Gooren L, Megens J. An epidemiological and demographic study of transsexuals in the Netherlands. *Arch Sex Behavior* 1996;25:589–600.

18. Jackson G, Rosen RC, Kloner RA, *et al*. The second Princeton Consensus on Sexual Dysfunction and Cardiac Risk: new guidelines for sexual medicine. *J Sex Med* 2006;3:28–36.

19. Giuliano F. Impact of medical treatments for benign prostatic hyperplasia on sexual function. *BJU Int* 2006;97(Suppl 2):34–8.

20. Grimm RH Jr, Grandits GA, Prineas RJ, *et al*. Long-term effects on sexual function of five antihypertensive drugs and nutritional hygienic treatment in hypertensive men and women. Treatment of mild hypertension study (TOMHS). *Hypertension* 1997;29(1, Pt 1):8–14.

21. de Tejada IS, Angulo J, Cellek S, *et al*. Pathophysiology of erectile dysfunction. *J Sex Med* 2005;2:26–39.

22. Jackson G, Betteridge J, Dean J, *et al.* A systematic approach to erectile dysfunction in the cardiovascular patient: a Consensus Statement – update 2002. *Int J Clin Pract* 2002;56:663–71.

23. Feldman HA, Goldstein I, Hatzichristou DG, *et al.* Impotence and its medical and psychosocial correlates: Results of the Massachusetts Male Aging Study. *J Urol* 1994;151:54–61.

24. Morales A, Buvat J, Gooren LJ, *et al.* Endocrine aspects of sexual dysfunction in men. *J Sex Med* 2004;1:69–81.

25. Wheeler MJ. Measurement of androgens. *Methods Mol Biol* 2006;324:197–211.

26. Vermeulen A, Verdonck L, Kaufman JM. A critical evaluation of simple methods for the estimation of free testosterone in serum. *J Clin Endocrinol Metab* 1999;84:3666–72.

27. Morley JE. Clinical diagnosis of age-related testosterone deficiency. *Aging Male* 2000;3(Suppl 1):195.

28. Heineman, LAJ, Saad F, Thiele K, *et al.* The aging male's symptom rating scale: Cultural and linguistic validation into English. *Aging Male* 2001;4:14–9.

29. Buvat J, Lemaire A, Buvat-Herbaut M, *et al.* Hyperprolactinemia and sexual function in men. *Horm Res* 1985;22:196–201.

30. Althof SE, Leiblum, SR, Chevret-Measson M, *et al.* Psychological and Interpersonal Dimensions of Sexual Function and Dysfunction. *J Sex Med* 2005;2:793–800.

31. Seidman SN. Roose SP, Menza MA, *et al.* Treatment of erectile dysfunction in men with depressive symptoms: results of a placebo-controlled trial with sildenafil citrate. *Am J Psychiatry* 2001;158:1623–30.

32. Costabile RA, Steers WD. How can we best characterize the relationship between erectile dysfunction and benign prostatic hyperplasia? *J Sex Med* 2006;3:676–81.

33. Eri LM, Tveter KJ. Safety, side effects and patient acceptance of the antiandrogen Casodex in the treatment of benign prostatic hyperplasia. *Eur Urol* 1994;26:219–26.

34. Mulhall J, Land S, Parker M, *et al.* The use of an erectogenic pharmacotherapy regimen following radical prostatectomy improves recovery of spontaneous erectile function. *J Sex Med* 2005;2:532–40.

35. Zelefsky MJ, Wallner KE, Ling CC, *et al.* Comparison of the 5-year outcome and morbidity of three-dimensional conformal radiotherapy versus transperineal permanent iodine-125 implantation for early-stage prostatic cancer. *J Clin Oncol* 1999;17:517–22.

36. Rabbani F, Stapleton AM, Kattan MW, *et al.* Factors predicting recovery of erections after radical prostatectomy. *J Urol* 2000;164:1929–34.

37. Kim NK, Aahn TW, Park JK, *et al.* Assessment of sexual and voiding function after total mesorectal excision with pelvic autonomic nerve preservation in males with rectal cancer. *Dis Colon Rectum* 2002;45:1178–85.

38. Kadioglu A, Oktar T, Kandirali E, *et al.* Incidentally diagnosed Peyronie's disease in men presenting with erectile dysfunction. *Int J Impot Res* 2004;16:540–3.

39. Ralph D. The surgical treatment of Peyronie's disease. *Eur Urol* 2006;50:196–8.

40. Leibovitch I, Mor Y. The vicious cycling: bicycling related urogenital disorders. *Eur Urol* 2005;47:277–86.

41. Derby CA, Mohr BA, Goldstein I, *et al.* Modifiable risk factors and erectile dysfunction: can lifestyle changes modify risk? *Urology* 2000;56:302–6.

42. Fisher WA, Rosen RC, Eardley I, *et al.* Sexual experience of female partners of men with erectile dysfunction: the Female Experience of Men's Attitudes to Life Events and Sexuality (FEMALES) Study. *J Sex Med* 2005;2:675–84.

43. Wagner G, Bondil P, Dabees K, *et al.* Ethical aspects of sexual medicine. *J Sex Med* 2005;2:163–8.

44. Riley A, Riley E. Behavioural and clinical findings in couples where the man presents with erectile disorder: a retrospective study. *Int J Clin Pract* 2000;54:220–4.

45. Dean J, de Boer B-J, Graziottin A, *et al.* Partner satisfaction and successful treatment

outcomes for men with erectile dysfunction (ED). *Eur Urol* 2006;(Suppl 5):779–85.

46. Dean J, de Boer B-J, Graziottin A, *et al*. The role of erection hardness in determining erectile dysfunction (ED) treatment outcome. *Eur Urol* 2006;(Suppl 5):767–72.

47. McCullough AR. Achieving treatment optimization with sildenafil citrate (Viagra) in patients with erectile dysfunction. *Urology* 2002;60(2, Suppl 2):28–38.

48. FDA-approved label for Viagra (sildenafil citrate). June, 2006.

49. FDA-approved label for Cialis (tadalafil). July, 2006.

50. FDA-approved label for Levitra (vardenafil). July, 2006.

51. Pavone C, Curto F, Anello G, *et al*. Prospective, randomized, crossover comparison of sublingual apomorphine (3 mg) with oral sildenafil (50 mg) for male erectile dysfunction. *J Urol* 2004;172(6, Pt 1):2347–9.

52. Turner LA, Althof SE, Levine SB, *et al*. Treating erectile dysfunction with external vacuum devices. *J Urol* 1990;144:79–82.

53. Meinhardt W, Lycklama a Nijeholt AA, *et al*. The negative pressure device for erectile disorders: when does it fail. *J Urol* 1993;149:1285–7.

54. Hatzichristou D, Moysidis K, Apostolidis A, *et al*. Sildenafil failures may be due to inadequate patient instructions and follow-up: a study on 100 non-responders. *Eur Urol* 2005;47:518–22.

55. Gruenwald I, Shenfeld O, Chen J, *et al*. Positive effect of counselling and dose adjustment in patients with erectile dysfunction who failed treatment with sildenafil. *Eur Urol* 2006;50:134–40.

56. McMahon C. Efficacy and safety of daily tadalafil in men with erectile dysfunction previously unresponsive to on demand tadalafil. *J Sex Med* 2004;1:292–300.

57. Eardley I. Optimisation of PDE5 inhibitor therapy in men with erectile dysfunction: converting 'non-responders' into 'responders'. *Eur Urol* 2006;50:31–3.

58. Montorsi F, Guazzoni G, Strambi LF, *et al*. Recovery of spontaneous erectile function after nerve-sparing radical radical retropubic prostatectomy with and without early intracavernous injections of alprostadil: results of a prospective, randomised trial. *J Urol* 1997;158:1408–10.

59. Mulhall J, Land S, Parker M, *et al*. The use of an erectogenic pharmacotherapy regimen following radical prostatectomy improves recovery of spontaneous erectile function. *J Sex Med* 2005;2:532–42.

60. FDA-approved label for Caverject (alprostadil). November, 2002.

61. Virag R. Intracavernous injection of papaverine for erectile failure. *Lancet* 1982;2:918.

62. Mulcahy JJ, Austoni E, Barada JH, *et al*. The penile implant for erectile dysfunction. *J Sex Med* 2004;1:98–109.

63. Carson CC, Mulcahy JJ, Govier FE. Efficacy, safety and patient satisfaction outcomes of the AMS 700CX inflatable penile prosthesis: results of a long-term multicenter study. AMS 700CX Study Group. *J Urol* 2000;164:376–80.

INDEX

Page references to figures and tables are shown in italics.